1001 littl
wellbeing mir

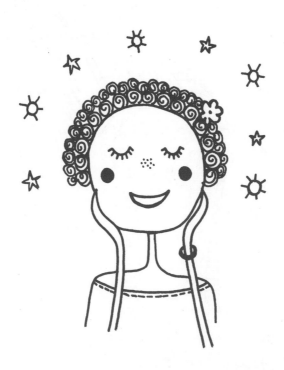

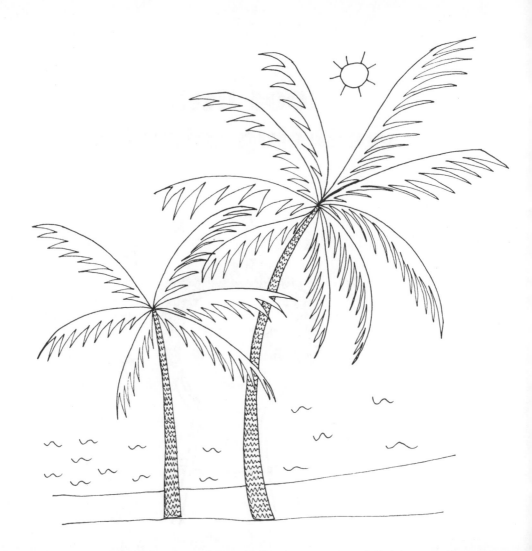

1001 little wellbeing miracles

Esme Floyd

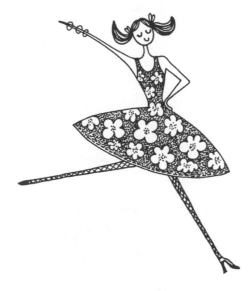

CARLTON
BOOKS

THIS IS A CARLTON BOOK

Text and design copyright © Carlton Books
Limited 2008

This edition published by
Carlton Books Limited
20 Mortimer Street
London W1T 3JW

10 9 8 7 6 5 4 3 2 1

A CIP catalogue record for this book is
available from the British Library.

ISBN 978 1 84732 146 6

Printed and bound in Dubai

Senior Executive Editor: Lisa Dyer
Managing Art Director: Lucy Coley
Designer: Zoë Dissell
Production: Kate Pimm

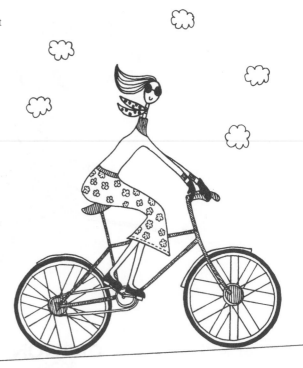

CONTENTS

INTRODUCTION

Did you know that laughing regularly could make you less prone to heart disease? Or that tidying up before you go to bed could help you sleep better?

From tips for organizing your home and office to getting your finances on track, changing bad habits and simply making you feel like a better you, this book contains 1001 little marvels to show you how small changes can make massive differences to your quality of life. The tips, which have been sourced from experts around the world, are astonishingly easy to follow, making this a must-have book for anyone who wants to have a happier and more serene life.

Top ten little wellbeing miracles

25
CLEAN LITTLE BY LITTLE
(see Happy home, page 15)

164
LISTENING SKILLS
(see Communication, page 49)

185
GET A LIFE BALANCE
(see Managing your lifestyle, page 56)

341
RESCUE YOURSELF
(see Natural remedies,
page 91)

507
KNOW YOUR SYMPTOMS
(see Depression, page 125)

553
KEEP IT REGULAR
(see Sleeping soundly, page 136)

602
GET ACTIVE
(see Harnessing happiness,
page 147)

698
HAVE A LAUGH
(see Laughter,
page 165)

796
DITCH THE BAGGAGE
(see Thirties, page 185)

995
HELP THEM FOCUS
(see Parenting,
page 213)

family favourites

1 FIVE A DAY

To help your family get their five portions of fruit and vegetables a day, encourage them to snack on fruit by having a bowl full of ready-washed fruit within easy reach. Keep the blender to hand and mix up smoothies in the morning – even those family members who are tempted to skip breakfast will have time for a drink.

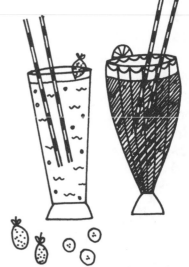

GET OUTSIDE

Walking is not only great exercise, it's often a really good time to have conversations about feelings and other issues. Borrow a dog for weekends or family walks, or go it alone and just enjoy nature.

SHARE THE CHORES

Make sure everyone in the house has a share in the chores. Even children as young as two or three can take some responsibility for tidying their toys, and taking a share of the housework makes everyone appreciate their home more.

DON'T EAT ALONE

If you live alone, try to eat with friends as often as you can to boost social happiness. Eating as a family is important to cement relationships, while in shared accommodation, make an effort to eat with housemates (even if you don't eat the same thing).

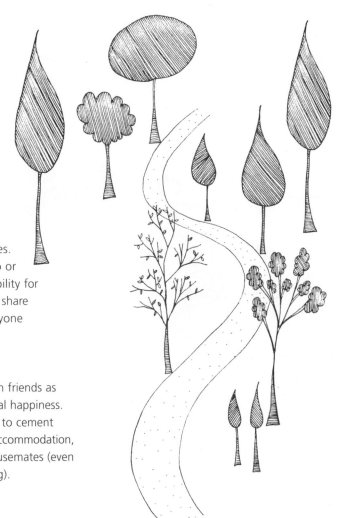

5 GO ON AN OUTING

Spend time with your family just doing something you all enjoy, like walking or visiting a park or museum, even going to the cinema or out for a meal to get to know what really makes them tick.

6 SET A TIMER

To help your children learn to share and to prevent stressful battles in the home, invest in an alarm you can set for 5 or 10 minutes so they know when their turn has finished.

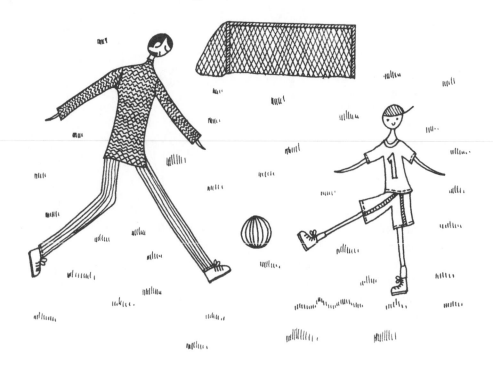

7 GET ROUTINE

Creating a routine for your children, especially around bedtime, will not only help them to settle down more easily, it will give you more time to help tie up those loose household ends.

8 BANK ONLINE

Moving your banking to online or telephone banking means you can avoid time-consuming trips to stand in the queue at the bank. Do as much of your banking as possible that way to help free up time.

9 COOK IT UP

Try to cook meals that will last more than one day. For instance, stews could be served one night with potato and the next with rice, or meat could be hot one night and cold with salad the next.

10 MAKE YOUR OWN

Instead of buying your coffee and snack on the way to work, take in your own and make it yourself. Not only will this save you time, you'll be amazed what a difference one coffee a day makes to your finances.

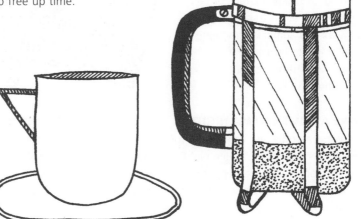

11 BOARD IT UP

Instead of gathering around the TV, encourage your family to relax by playing cards or a board game, which will help you spend quality time being engaged with each other.

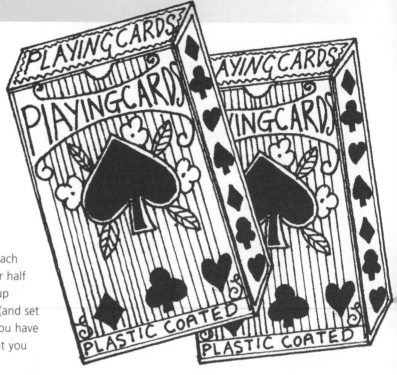

12 SET A TIMETABLE

Have a set homework time each evening. Set aside an hour or half an hour and use it to catch up on work and administration (and set an example to your kids, if you have them). Make it public, so that you won't be disturbed.

13 HAVE A HOME CINEMA NIGHT

Every few months, get your family together and have a real home cinema night. Choose a movie together, make popcorn or home-made pizza and enjoy watching and talking about a film. In the summer, why not set up a screen and move outdoors?

14 MAKE JOINT DECISIONS

When it comes to big issues like where to go on holiday or what to do with the house, let your children be involved and respect their input. Working together as a team to make decisions will help them develop cooperative social skills.

happy home

15 GO GREEN FINGERED

One of the easiest ways to make your home feel like a healthier environment is to include house plants, particularly in areas you spend a lot of time in. Choose plants you like the look of and never keep dead plants.

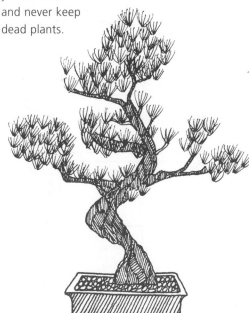

16 MAKE A STATEMENT

Don't fall into the trap of not reading your bank statements. Not only is it important to check each transaction thoroughly to ensure you are protected against fraud, it will also help you to stay on top of spending.

17 STOCK UP

Make a point of keeping a stock of certain basics you need for organizing your home or home office. That way, you won't have to pop to the store every time you need them. Stamps, envelopes, notepaper and pens are all good staple choices.

18 MAKE YOUR BED

Making your bed when you leave the house in the morning might sound a strange way to help yourself cope better with life, but starting the day organized is a great way to stay positive for longer. Taking a few minutes to smooth down those sheets every morning could actually help you off to a better start to the day.

19 ENJOY YOUR HOME

Don't make your home a place only of chores and 'to do' lists. Make an effort to enjoy spending time there doing something that makes you feel happy, relaxed and refreshed.

20 FILE A BILL

Make a habit of keeping receipts and bills together so it's easy to arrange your finances and check bank statements. This will also save you hours when it's time to get your taxes filed.

21 CATCH UP AT THE WEEKEND

Weekends are for enjoyment but they are also a great chance to get set for the next week. Spend a few hours making sure you have work clothes, food for lunches, etc, ready for Monday morning.

22 STICK TO IT

Don't give up if your attempts at managing your time better don't work immediately. It takes a while to learn good habits, so stick to it until it works.

23 GET RID OF PILES

Go through those piles of papers on your desk that have been sitting there for ever, file the important documents and shred the rest. Then work out a system to stop the papers piling up again and stick to it.

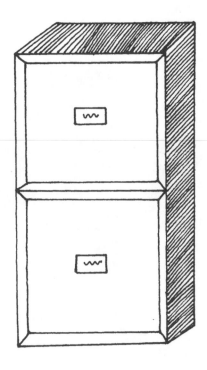

24 DIG YOURSELF HAPPY

Gardening has long been hailed as a way to help ease problems and reduce stress hormones. Because it combines fresh air – which boosts mood as well as improving vitamin levels – with low-level exercise, it helps the brain unwind. Aim for 30 minutes two or three times a week.

25 CLEAN LITTLE BY LITTLE

There's nothing worse than having the week's cleaning or household organization hanging over you all week. Instead of leaving it all to the weekend, or your one particular time a week, clean small areas regularly. Doing a little bit each day will keep it more manageable, help you to stay relaxed and ultimately save time.

26 DITCH THE OFFICE

Never allow computers or work into your bedroom. It should be a space devoted to sleep and relaxation, and a place to be together with your partner for intimacy, not a place to be reminded of work.

27 DO A SPRING CLEAN

It might sound like a cliché, but devoting a weekend to giving your house a spring clean will help your mind feel fresh as a daisy, too. Do it in spring when the light starts to increase and you can see the dirt.

28 GO SOFT

One of the best investments you can make for your bedroom is to make sure you choose sheets that are soft and made of natural fabrics that allow your skin to breathe. This will help enhance deep, healing sleep and help you feel better through the day.

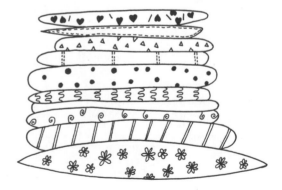

29 DO A DANCE

The old myth about dancing while you do the housework is really true – dancing does make you happier, so turn up the volume and get grooving (and you'll have a clean house, too!).

30 LIMIT YOUR SCREEN TIME

Don't allow yourself to slump in front of the TV for hours every night, which can actually make you feel more lethargic. Instead, limit yourself to certain TV times and use the rest to achieve something.

31 BUY A ROBE

A great way to enhance the feeling of relaxation in your home is to invest in a really luxurious bathrobe. Don't make it your everyday robe; save it for your special relaxation times to mark the difference.

32 REFLECT IN YOUR HOME

One of the best ways to spruce up your home environment in just a few minutes is to give your windows and mirrors a clean. Not only will it improve light levels, it will make the whole place look and feel cleaner. Large clean mirrors are also good feng shui, bringing calm and refreshment while reflecting away negativity.

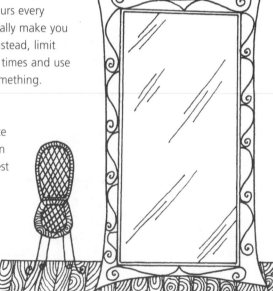

decluttering

33 GET ENVIRONMENTAL

Take a good look at the various different environments you spend time in – your home, workplace and friends' or family's houses – and ask yourself if they are positive, negative or neutral places. What can you do to make them more positive? Making a list can help.

34 DON'T BE A SQUARE

Your mother used to joke that watching TV would give you square eyes, but nowadays it's more likely to be the computer screen you're staring at for hours. Don't allow yourself more than a few hours a day in front of any screen during leisure time.

35 KEEP THEM HAPPY

Don't forget that everyone in your home will benefit from a bit of pampering. Next time you treat yourself, get a little something for everyone else in the house as well to enhance the feeling of wellbeing (and that includes the pets!). It doesn't have to be much but if the thought is there, it will be appreciated.

36 HAVE A CHARITY MONTH

Do you feel overwhelmed by the sheer amount of stuff in your home? For one month, put away one thing every day to take to the charity shop. Not only will you be helping local charities but your house will be much less cluttered.

37 ONE IN ONE OUT

To solve serious storage problems, develop a 'one-in one-out' system where for every new thing you accumulate you have to get rid of something. You'll be amazed how many new things slip by unnoticed unless you pay attention. It could save you money, too.

38 MAKE A DIVIDE

Divide your wardrobe into winter and summer clothes and make sure at the end of each season that clothes are cleaned, ironed and put away. This will free up storage space and help you ring the changes.

39 DECLUTTER

There's nothing more irritating than a
room with clutter in it. Try to develop
a storage system where everything has
a place to reduce those 'moving from
place to place' clutter problems. Stock
items neatly on shelves and they will be
more pleasurable to look at and use.

40 DON'T BE A HOARDER

If the sight of your overcrowded
wardrobe (closet) makes you run for
cover, develop a clothes system – each
season, put away clothes you won't
wear until the next, and give or throw
away anything you haven't worn for
more than six months.

41 DE-JUNK YOUR LIFE

It's hard to be happy unless you can
think clearly, and it's hard to think
clearly if you're living in a clutter bomb.
Make it a rule to have a clear-out a
couple of times a year and sell, give
away, recycle or throw out anything
you're unlikely to use.

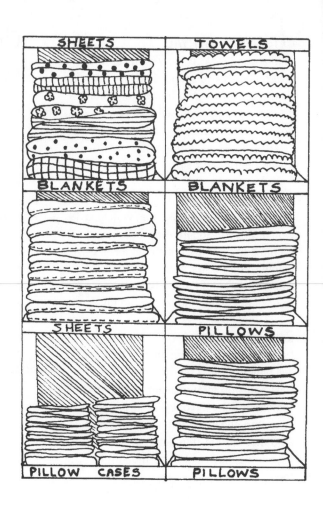

42 CLEANSE YOUR MIND

Give your mind a cleanse as well as your body and home. Invest in a book of meditations for your bathroom. Before you take a bath or shower read just one of them, and use your time in the bath or shower to think about the words and what they mean.

43 PLAY IT AGAIN

One of the best ways to turn your home into a place for relaxation is through music. Play some of your favourite tunes and allow yourself to really listen to them without any distractions.

44 CULL YOUR FILES

Do you really need to keep every birthday card you've been given since you were a kid, or every bank statement since you opened your account? Keep financial documents for six years and get rid of as much of the rest as you can.

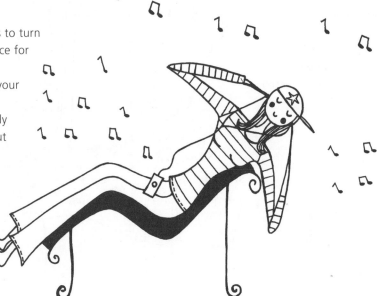

creating a sanctuary

45 WATER DOWN YOUR MOODS

Adding a water feature to your room, balcony, patio or garden is a great happiness booster. It is thought that the sound of running water penetrates deep into our subconscious, helping the brain rid itself of stress.

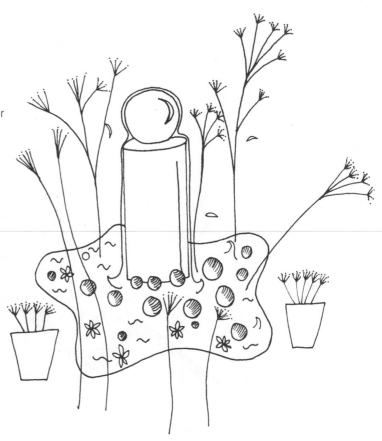

46 GET COLOURFUL

Changing the colour of your bedroom walls can give the room a completely new feel, and help you to relax inside it. Try soft blues or greens to create a relaxing space; just paint one wall if you don't like too much colour. If you don't want to paint the walls, try incorporating artwork and wall-hangings that feature those colours to help relax your mood.

47 CHOOSE NATURAL MATERIALS

Invite nature into your home by choosing natural fabrics and colours. Choose wood, wicker, cotton and earthy tones as well as blues and greens to help you reconnect with the world outside. Maximize comfort levels – soft sheets, pretty cushions, pillows you can sink into, and a variety of textures and colours all aid relaxation.

48 LIGHT A CANDLE

Candlelight is of a lower luminescence than electric light and so our eyes find it easier to stay relaxed by the warmer glow of candles. Use them in your bathroom or while you eat. It will help you stay relaxed and calm.

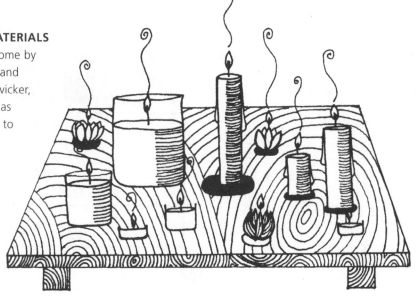

49 GET LUXURIOUS

Luxury doesn't have to break the bank, and it will help you feel more relaxed and pampered in your own home. Collect old perfume bottles to store your toiletries and choose silk and satin for an opulent feel.

50 STAY CLOSE

Help your sanctuary become a 'you' space by keeping photos of your friends and family close to hand. If you don't want them on display, keep an album available and flick through it when you need to centre yourself.

51 STRIKE A LIGHT

Take a look at the light levels around your house at different times of day and choose to spend time in rooms with the best light. For instance, maybe your bedroom is best for morning relaxation but the kitchen has better light in the evening.

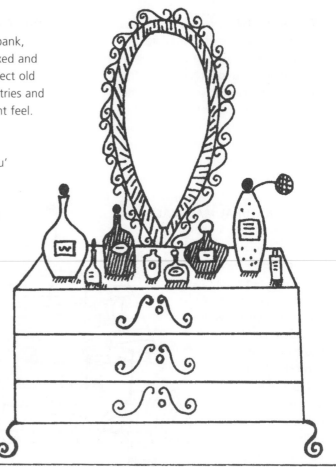

52 GO HOME

At the end of a busy day, take at least 5 or 10 minutes before your evening begins just to sit or lie down in the quiet of your house or apartment. If your space is noisy, use earplugs to help you stay tranquil.

53 ITCHY FEET

Instead of slumping in front of the television or going out with friends every night, make one night a week your 'self improvement' night. Use it to further your skills in whatever area you'd like to develop – whether it be a new language or hobby.

54 KEEP THINGS NEAT

Making your bed every morning and tidying up clothes dropped on the floor will help your bedroom feel like a retreat rather than a hovel. Try to keep surfaces as clean as possible and don't allow clutter to build up.

55 BE SINGLE-MINDED

The bedroom is the most important room to keep for single use – that of sleeping. If you truly want better sleep and relaxation, don't put a computer or television in the bedroom.

56 IT'S ELEMENTAL

Make your living area more relaxing by enlivening it with natural elements, such as stone and water. According to feng shui, an aquarium combines water and living energy (*chi*), which stimulates energy and brings good luck and wealth.

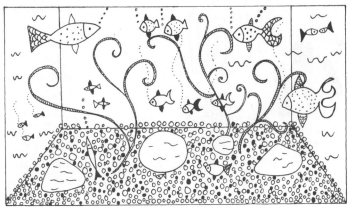

getting organized

57 DARN THE TV

Keep a sewing kit in your living room near the television so you can make essential repairs while you're watching something interesting. It will make you more likely to do the job rather than letting the mending pile mount up.

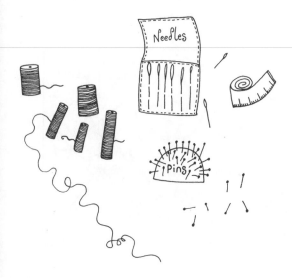

58 MAKE A LIST

If your life requires multitasking, stay on top of your different responsibilities by taking a few minutes every morning to make a list of everything that needs to be done in each of your life areas. Tick them off as you go along so that you never lose track of what needs doing, and update it the next day.

59 KEEP A WORKBOOK

Keep all your handy telephone numbers in one place – such as plumber, builder, car garage or repair services – and use the same place to make a note of serial numbers, guarantee numbers, etc, of your items, so you have everything you need when you need to make the call.

60 GET FIRE RESISTANT

Keep your important documents, like passports, birth certificates and insurance policies, inside a flame-retardant box so you won't have to worry about losing them. Irreplaceable documents should be kept with a lawyer or at a bank, with a copy at home for reference.

61 REMEMBER BIRTHDAYS

Make a birthday calendar and keep it
in a prominent place, in your home
office or in the kitchen. Look at
it every week to make sure
you're not forgetting
important events, which
could make you feel bad.

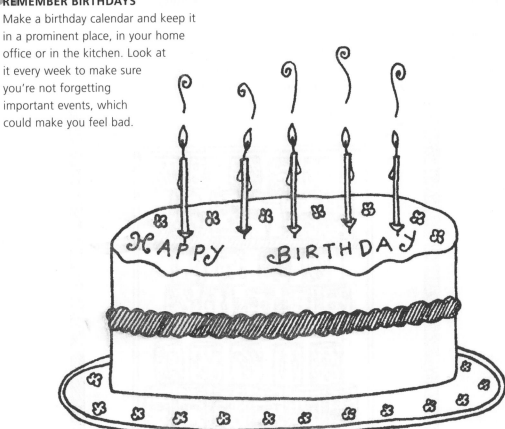

62 GET REGULAR

Clean one cupboard a week rather than leaving it all to one mammoth job, which could pile up and cause stress. That way, your house will feel as if it's being constantly cleaned with little effort for you.

63 BE PREPARED

Always keep a few essentials like bread, milk and butter in the deep freeze so you can be sure you're protected in case of emergency. You never know when they might be useful and it will put your mind at rest.

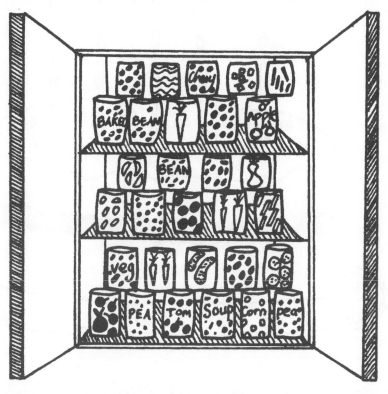

64 SEE DOUBLE

Why not have two laundry baskets – one for whites and one for colours? It will save you masses of time sorting out the washing loads, and you'll never have to worry about colours running again!

65 GET MULTIPLE

Buy enough essential clothes items like underwear and socks for a couple of weeks so you don't have to worry about running out or rushing to do the washing.

66 TIDY AT NIGHT

Before you go to sleep, make sure you spend a few minutes tidying away your shoes or putting dirty clothes into the laundry basket so that when you wake up in the morning the first thing you see is an orderly room.

67 KEY TO SUCCESS

Make a place for your keys so you don't keep misplacing them. Make it prominent but not too near the front or back door (which could give burglars an easy way to make their escape).

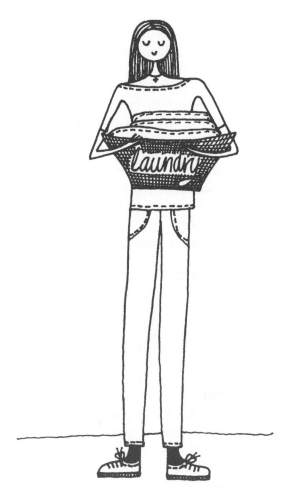

27

68 ON-THE-SPOT NOTEBOOK

Keep a notebook or a pad stuck to the fridge or on the wall in the kitchen so you can make a note of anything you've run out of. Encourage everyone in the house to use it so you don't have to remember everything.

69 TAKE A COURSE

If you feel your life is constantly escaping from under your feet and you simply don't have time to do anything, think about doing a time-management course, which could help you see things differently.

70 PLAN YOUR DRESS

If you find your clothes are often in chaos, why not spend a few weeks sticking to a clothing plan. Work out what you're going to wear in advance and make sure you have enough for a two-week cleaning rotation.

71 SLEEP IT OUT

Studies have shown that couples who get enough sleep are generally happier than those who don't, so make your bedroom work for both of you.

72 MAKE AN EXIT

Decide on a realistic time to leave work every day – for instance, if you know you always need to stay later on Wednesdays, be honest about it, but make sure you leave earlier on other days. Stick to your times to help you leave work behind at night.

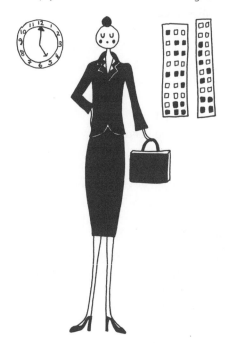

73 ORGANIZE YOUR HOME

Don't leave important home phone calls, like paying bills and organizing visits, to chance. Free up an hour a week where you can sit down with your diary and phone numbers and organize your home life so important tasks aren't left undone.

74 ASK FOR HELP

Don't hide your head in the sand. There's nothing worse than feeling as if you've got too much on your plate and things are out of control. You're much more likely to be able to get yourself out of the situation by facing up to it and asking for help.

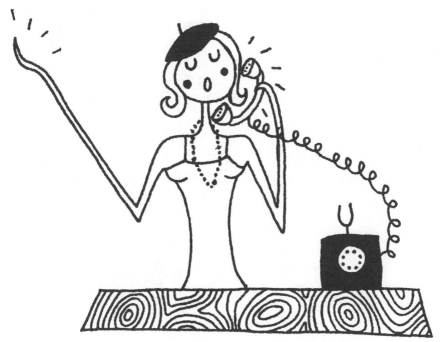

enjoying life

75 CLEAR YOUR HEAD

If you're trying to get your head around a problem, taking the time to go for a walk or a run – or simply to have a bath if you prefer – can give you valuable subconscious insight. Don't think about the problem deliberately; just give your brain space to process and you'll be amazed at the solutions that spring to mind.

76 EAT EARLY

Skipping breakfast, which leads to low blood sugar in the morning, can play havoc with memory and concentration. To help you start the day thinking straight, make sure you eat something nutritious.

77 GET MUSICAL

Listen to relaxing music while travelling through the city. Driving or even walking in a busy city can be stressful, and listening to light, calming music will help you to keep your inner calm among the whirlwind of people and cars.

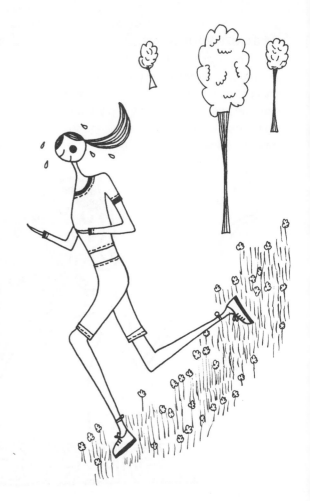

78 MAKE GOOD DECISIONS

If you've got a big decision to make, such as whether to move house or change jobs, it's imperative to write a list of goals. Make note of everything that's important to you and what your priorities are, including those of your partner, and make a decision that works towards them.

79 GO BY THE LIST

Be flexible and realistic when planning your day. Work through your list in order of priority and don't allow yourself to be distracted – it will help you feel in control of your day rather than it being in control of you.

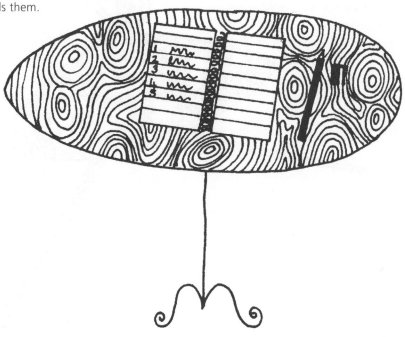

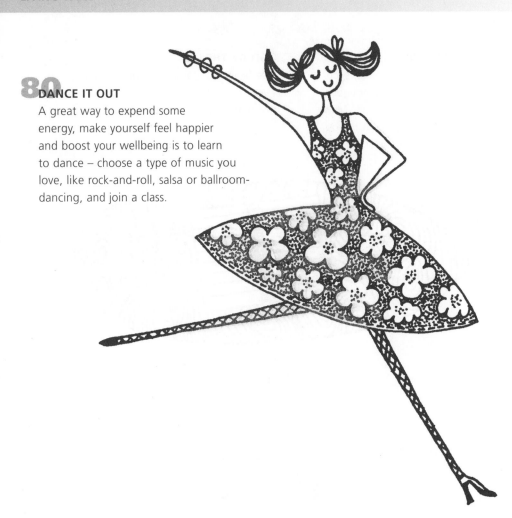

80 DANCE IT OUT

A great way to expend some
energy, make yourself feel happier
and boost your wellbeing is to learn
to dance – choose a type of music you
love, like rock-and-roll, salsa or ballroom-
dancing, and join a class.

81 BACK TO NATURE

Spend time at the nearest park, tree-lined path, river, lake or beach whenever possible. Being in nature, even if it is bang in the middle of a buzzing city, is calming and restorative. It will help you to relax.

82 BE A BOOKWORM

Read a book while taking public transport through a city. Choose books that are funny, relaxing or calming so that you can get your mind off your commute and lose yourself in your book.

83 MAKE A CHANGE

Change is refreshing, so do something different at least once a month. This could be something big like trying a new adventure sport or going away for the weekend, or something small like taking a new route for your daily walk or visiting a different pub.

84 TAKE A BREAK

If you work in a city, it's even more important to take small breaks throughout the day. Step outside the office, even if only for 5 minutes, to breathe deeply, look at the sky and step out of the mayhem for a few minutes.

85 REMEMBER TO RELAX

Don't fall into the trap of scheduling your whole life into activity slots. Make sure you incorporate leisure and relaxation time for yourself when planning your schedule and stick to it as rigidly as you would to your other time slots.

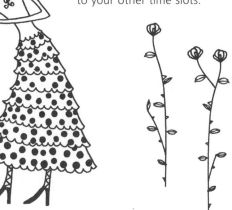

relationships

86 BE APPRECIATIVE

Learn to do the one thing that is most likely
to restore good feeling in your relationship
– giving your partner a genuine, loving and
approving smile. A simple hug, too, can
help restore contact and affection without
even having to say a word.

87 INVEST IN QUALITY

Without quality time, your relationship
will not survive. Carve out at least half
an hour a night and at least one day a
month when the two of you spend time
exclusively together. Talk to each other
and make a pact not to bring up problems
or arguments during these times.

88 LEARN TO COMPROMISE

A good relationship is built on compromise
on both sides. Choose three things each
that you feel you really can't compromise
on and agree to work with each other on
those areas, then be willing to give way
on the other, less significant, things.

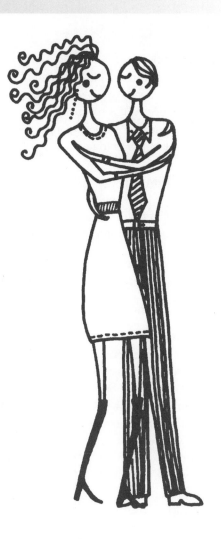

89 DON'T BE CODEPENDENT

Keep your dependence and independence in balance. Tell and show your partner how much you need them, but don't cling or try to control them as that can make your partner feel trapped.

90 LEND AN EAR

Encourage your partner to listen to you by showing appreciation when they do and make an effort to let yourself hear what your partner is saying rather than assuming you know what's coming next.

91 ANGER OR BOREDOM?

Remember that boredom typically covers up anger so if you're feeling bored with your partner or with your life, ask yourself what you're angry about.

92 GO OUT

Make an effort to see your friends without your partner as often as you can, preferably once a month. It will remind you of the 'you' that's inside, independent of partners, jobs and families.

93 TEACH EACH OTHER

Don't be shy about what you want in the bedroom – save the guesswork and teach your partner (preferably early on in the relationship) exactly what you need to feel satisfied. Just don't forget to be prepared to hear the same from them.

94 MAKE SOME SPACE

Don't assume your partner needs the same things as you when you're arguing or tense. You might want to talk, but many people need some 'space' to get their heads straight. Being understanding about what your partner needs will lead to a more fruitful discussion in the long run.

95 LIST THE GOOD THINGS

When your relationship feels really good, such as after a great meal out, or when you feel things are going well, take the time to write down what makes you love your partner so much and why you're with them. Referring back to it during the bad times or a rocky patch may help you get some perspective.

96 SET THE TIMER

If you've got a issue that needs discussing, try a mediator's timing method to help clarify both sides of the argument. Set the timer for 5 minutes and take turns talking – the only rule is that during your 5 minutes your partner is not allowed to interrupt, and vice versa.

97 FORGET PERFECTION

Nobody's perfect, and it's unreasonable of you to expect your partner not to have bad habits just like everyone else. Don't try to change them too much because chances are it won't work; instead, try to love them warts and all.

98 COMPLIMENT YOURSELF

If your partner is bad at giving compliments, instead of letting your resentment build up, make them appreciate you. Say something good about yourself and ask for their agreement – it will encourage them to think of nice things to say.

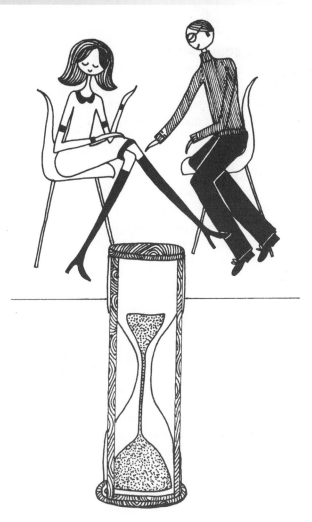

99 OUT IN THE OPEN

Hidden resentments poison a relationship so if something is bothering you, say it. But don't nag or assign blame; simply express the problem as you see it and ask your partner to help you find the answer. That way, you're working together and nobody feels blamed.

100 NEVER SAY NEVER

When you have a disagreement or argument, avoid the phrases 'you never ...' and 'you always ...' They are rarely true and inevitably cause defensive reactions, which won't help you to move forward. Even if they are true, saying them is unlikely to lead to the person changing.

101 THINK FIRST

Next time your partner tries to tell you something negative about yourself, make an effort not to respond immediately. It's tempting to jump to your own defence, but instead, try really listening to what they've got to say and let them finish before you bite back.

102 BE A NEGOTIATOR

Set a rule that each of you states what you want and then both of you work together to find a way forward. If you really work together, no problem is unsolvable.

103 A DUAL PARENT

If you have children, involve your partner as much as possible with the child care, even if you feel they are not as good at it or as natural as you are. It's important to present a united front to your children.

104 DON'T BANK ON SUCCESS

Money is the number-one cause of couple conflict. For a relationship to work, you need to address your finances and work out a budget. Be honest about debt and spending, and come to a joint solution.

105 END OF THE AFFAIR

If you do stray, don't feel it necessarily spells the end of your relationship. Most couples recover and some find that unearthing the cause of the affair helps them get closer.

106 DON'T FAN THE BLAME

Learning how to argue well is an art. Try to avoid using blame words like 'you make me …' and opt for softer versions like 'when you …, it makes me feel …' instead.

107 BALANCE THE PAIN

Think about your relationship in terms of balance. If there is consistently more pain than pleasure, more hurt than enjoyment or more arguments than laughter, then something's got to change.

108 BITE YOUR TONGUE

If you're arguing with your partner, keep one golden rule in mind – never say anything you wouldn't want said to you. That way, you'll learn to phrase your anxieties better and avoid causing hurt.

109 GET A BUNCH OF FIVE

Research suggests you need five positive experiences to erase the memory of one negative experience. So aim to give five kind words for each negative comment you give, even if done inadvertently.

110 DIVIDE AND RULE

If the domestic work is not divided fairly between you, it will cause friction in your relationship. Make a list of the domestic tasks, talk it through with your partner and mobilize the whole family, your partner included, to share the workload.

111 SORT THE SEX

Your sex life may ebb and flow over the years, but if the actual sex starts going downhill (rather than the frequency) don't accept it. As soon as you notice a slide, question why and work at bringing the passion back. Discuss with your partner what might be happening sooner rather than later and be honest with each other.

112 SEEK PROFESSIONAL HELP

Professional help can turn a bad relationship into a great one. Don't feel that seeing a professional counsellor, marriage guidance or sex therapist means you've failed – what it actually means is that you're taking steps to work things out together and it could save your relationship.

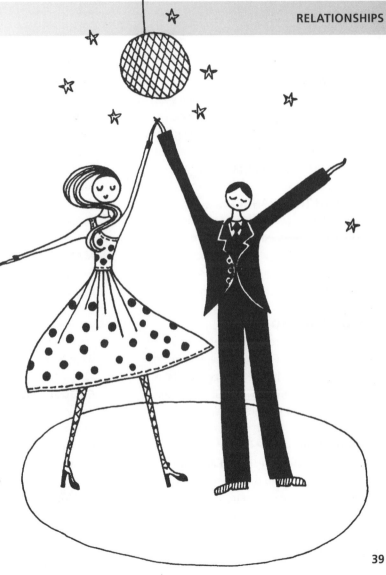

113 DANCE THE BLUES AWAY

Research has shown that couples who do some form of activity together – like dancing – are happier and more contented with each other than those who have separate interests. Choose a type of dancing that fits the music you like and enrol in a course to learn the basics.

114 GET TRAINING

Instead of nagging or moaning when your partner does something you don't like, ignore it and concentrate on the things they do that you do like. Positive reinforcement works much better than punishment.

115 GO WITH THE CHANGES

People change over the years so even if you think you understand you partner now, or believe you have agreements sorted, check regularly – at least once a year – to make sure neither of you has changed your mind.

116 KNOW WHEN TO QUIT

If your life aims are really incompatible and you feel you can't compromise, ending the relationship may be the only option. Take professional marital advice but don't feel you must stay if you aren't happy.

117 WRAP IT UP

Make your partner feel good and give yourself a boost too by writing a list of things you like about them, then giving it to them for no particular reason.

sex

118 TALK IT OUT

Talking about sex when you're stressed about it isn't easy but starting with a little tenderness will help. Ask your partner to hold you close and use that physical intimacy as a platform to talk about your sexual problems, worries or desires.

119 MAKE IT WORK

Good sex starts with love and affection, and part of ensuring you both have a good time is being honest. Don't be pressured by what you see in films or read in magazines, which are often invented anyway; tell each other what works for YOU.

120 CHOOSE YOUR WORDS

You want to ask your partner to do something differently in bed but you don't want it to sound like a criticism. Avoid using negative phrases like 'I don't like it when you …' and instead opt for positives such as 'I love it when …' or 'we could try …'. Don't expect it to all change overnight.

121 DON'T GET STUCK IN A RUT

Sex doesn't always have to be in the
bedroom – spontaneity can be really sexy,
so go for it in the kitchen, lounge, garden
or even on your Sunday
afternoon walk. Try new
sexy underwear or sex
toys to spark up your
love life, too.

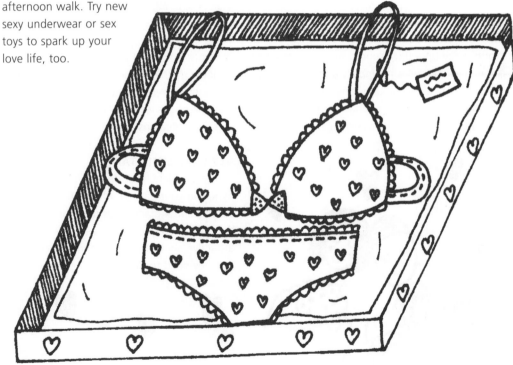

122 THE SOUND OF MUSIC

Use music to get you in the mood for sex. Make a playlist of your favourite tracks – and those of your partner – and play it to help aid relaxation, promote romance and bring back good memories.

123 GET TOUCHY FEELY

Words make up a tiny proportion of human communication, which is mostly done through body language and tone of voice. Back up your words with behaviour by touching and holding your partner.

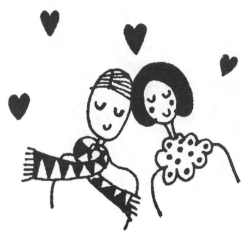

124 BE HONEST

If your partner does something that rocks your world next time you're having sex, don't assume they will realize it. Tell them you loved what they did and not only will it boost their ego, it might make it happen again!

125 TALK DIRTY

Feeling stressed and tired can make it difficult to get in the mood for sex, but talking about your fantasies can help change your mindset into one of desire. Share fantasies over dinner and then retire upstairs!

126 GET COMPLIMENTARY

Take your relationship to new heights by telling your partner what you love about them – many of us take for granted that our loved ones know what we find attractive about them, but the chances are they need to be told.

127 OPEN YOUR EYES

Many people make love with their eyes shut, particularly if they feel self-conscious in bed. Try doing it with your eyes open for a change and you may feel a higher level of intimacy.

128 BE GRATEFUL

Say thank you to your partner if they make you feel good in the bedroom – good sex is like giving and receiving a gift, so saying thank you is a great way to let them know it's appreciated.

129 HOLD YOUR TONGUE

Never make derisory comments about your partner's sexual performance. Ridiculing it or making them feel bad will only lead to insecurity, which will affect future performance. Be supportive.

130 BE A SOFT TOUCH

Use massage to help you relax before a sex session. Use light strokes which have been shown to stimulate the body's natural feel-good chemicals, or endorphins, and enjoy better sex as a result.

breaking up

131 ENJOY LIFE

After a relationship breakdown, help yourself see the positive side by treating yourself to all the things you like but your partner didn't. This will remind you of what you were giving up during the relationship and what you have now regained.

132 TIME TO GRIEVE

For most people, it's a shock when a relationship breaks down, even if you've known for some time that things weren't right. If your relationship ends, give yourself a few months of grieving time for the life you thought you would have.

133 FACE UP TO IT

Going through a divorce is a stressful time for everyone involved, all of whom can suffer damaging effects. The first step to helping you get through a breakup successfully is to acknowledge that these effects can't be fixed straight away. Healing takes time.

134 SEEK SUPPORT

Although it's tempting to cloister yourself from others, don't turn away offers of help and company if your relationship has just broken down. You might not feel like going out, but why not suggest spending time with friends at home instead.

135 STAY CLOSE TO FAMILY

Friends and family play a major role in helping you rebuild your life after a relationship split. Try to organize regular gatherings which can help you have some fun and get your life back on track. Ask your friends to organize them if you don't feel you can.

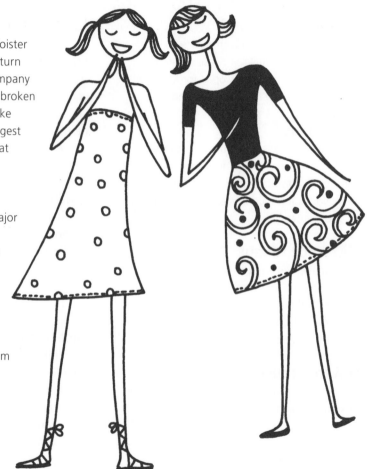

136 DREAMS AREN'T REAL

It's not unusual for people who are divorcing, or even those who have been divorced for a long time, to have dreams about their ex-spouse. Sometimes they're even good dreams or sexual in nature. It doesn't mean you harbour secret desires for reconciliation.

137 GET IN FOCUS

Don't just think about your individual problems when it comes to analyzing your relationship breakdown. Think about external factors too, and what changes you might be able to make to ensure future relationships are protected.

138 GIVE YOURSELF TIME

After a relationship breakdown, many people find themselves struggling with low self-esteem and confidence, and with so many things to organize – such as children and moving house – it can be hard to find time for your own feelings. Remember you need to look after yourself and give yourself some time to heal.

139 FORGIVE OR FORGET

If you know you will never forgive your partner over something important, then give them – and yourself – a break and start again, with someone else. But if you do say you forgive them, you have to mean it.

140 BE HONEST WITH CHILDREN

Don't try to hide the situation from your children if your relationship is ending. As a parent, it's natural to want to protect them but not being honest can leave them feeling confused.

141 ANSWER QUESTIONS

One of the best ways to talk to your children about a relationship breakup is to give them a brief explanation and then allow them to ask questions.

142 GAIN UNDERSTANDING

Understanding why a relationship failed is the first step to getting over it. Don't worry about whose fault it was, which isn't constructive. Instead concentrate on what stopped you overcoming your differences.

143 BE CARING

It's tough being a parent when you're splitting up, but understand that your children will need more care and reassurance than normal. Let them know they're loved and try to present a united front.

144 MAKE A CHOICE

How a person handles the sad reality of separating from a relationship is a matter of personal choice. Try to have the view that it is a learning experience rather than a failure.

145 SEEK ADVICE

It's normal to feel anxious and fearful when situations change, and especially if your relationship is ending, but you're not alone. Join a support group or seek advice from websites or organizations.

146 GET MEDIATION

If there are children involved in your relationship split and you don't think you can work together to come to an arrangement, getting a mediator involved can help cut out emotional arguments and reach a solution.

147 HAVE A CLEAROUT

If you're splitting up, clearing out your ex's belongings can help provide some closure. Holding on to items such as clothes, personal effects and memorabilia may only bring back painful memories, hindering the move to start anew.

148 FOCUS ON SUCCESS

It's difficult to keep your self-esteem high if you're going through a relationship breakdown. Although boosting self-confidence doesn't happen overnight, focusing on little successes rather than big failures can help. For example, give yourself a pat on the back for that DIY job you finished or that job application you made.

149 EXTEND A HAND

One of the major worries for children involved in separations is that they will lose contact with their extended family, particularly grandparents. Make an effort to include former in-laws and maintain contact with them so that your children feel supported.

150 THINK OF YOURSELF

If you're going through a stressful time, like a separation, it's easy to start obsessing about what other people might think of your situation. But this is not going to help you. Instead, try to focus on healing your own feelings.

151 KEEP A JOURNAL

Instead of wallowing in feelings of loneliness, use your energy to write down how you feel. Keep a notebook to hand and use it when you need to express something or when you're feeling bad. Even if you're writing about a negative feeling, the process can be positive and constructive.

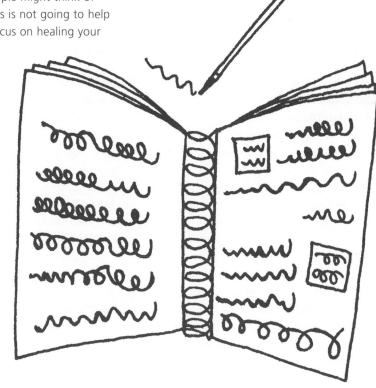

152 SEE A PROFESSIONAL

If things become too unbearable, don't be afraid to seek the help of a professional like a counsellor, church minister or psychiatrist. They will be able to help you see the situation from another angle without adding to your emotional burden, and they won't be giving advice based on whatever they might be going through, as friends might.

153 TALK IT THROUGH

If you've been separated for a while and suddenly start having feelings about your ex, don't feel you can't approach them to talk about it. Sometimes they'll be receptive, sometimes they won't, but perhaps an effective reconciliation can be made.

154 GET OVER IT

Not getting over a divorce can mean you haven't been able to take stock of yourself as an independent person but still see yourself as merged with that other person. After a period of grieving, make a decision to stop talking about your ex and the divorce and start thinking about yourself.

communication

155 PICK YOUR TIME

Don't try to initiate an important discussion when you're feeling low. Try to choose a time of day when you're likely to be feeling your best, and arrange to have the discussion then.

156 ARGUE WELL

A good rule of thumb for arguments is to make sure you stick to the point and don't drag in old grievances. If anyone starts to lose control, take time out to calm down and finish the discussion later.

157 TAKE CRITICISM WELL

Next time someone criticizes you, take a breath before you bite back and ask yourself, is it really a criticism and if it is, could there conceivably be a grain of truth in there?

158 LISTEN AND LEARN

Empathize by restating or rephrasing what's been said: Use phrases like 'it sounds as if …' or 'what I'm hearing is …', which will open the door to further discussion.

159 LISTEN TO YOURSELF FIRST

The starting point for all good communication is knowing what you want to say before you say it, and getting your point across in a way other people understand. Take a moment to listen to yourself before you speak.

160 THINK AHEAD

If you're trying to tell someone something important, practise first. Think of possible barriers to getting your point across, such as interruptions or questions, and how you will deal with them if they arise. It can help to clarify things in your own mind if you write things down first. Keep rewriting until you're happy about what you want to say and how you'll deal with barriers.

161 STAY CALM

You communicate most effectively when you're calm, so try to relax before the discussion, and do your best not to become emotional during the conversation. If you get heated, the other person may too, then neither of you will be very effective.

162 TAKE OFF THE HEAT

If things do start to get out of hand when you're trying to have a discussion, suggest that you continue the conversation later, when both of you are feeling less emotional about it. And do try to set a time and a place before you part.

163 USE 'I' MESSAGES

Let the other person know how you're feeling about the situation by using 'I messages' – statements that start with 'I feel ...' or 'I felt ...'. These are a stronger, positive way to start rather than 'you messages', which introduce blame and can provoke a hostile reaction.

164 LISTENING SKILLS

You might know exactly what you want to say if you're having a discussion with someone else, but discussion means just that – it's a two-way process. You've got to listen as well as saying your piece, and try to find a common ground. Stop yourself from jumping in with your opinion too quickly, and really listen to what's being said.

time savers

165 MAKE WORK WORK FOR YOU

If you don't enjoy your job but don't feel you have a choice about giving up for something else, don't fall into the trap of wasting your time. If you have to stay in your job, work hard and try to find a niche within it that suits you.

166 GIVE YOURSELF A KISS

Whenever you feel life's getting on top of you, remember the KISS principle – Keep It Simple, Stupid! Problems often crop up because we allow things to become overcomplicated, so keeping it simple is a great way to keep things in perspective. An approach that seems to easy to be true can be simply the best way.

167 LEAVE GAPS

When you plan your day, don't fill every minute. Leave about 15–20% for contingencies. Then, if emergencies and interruptions happen, you won't be thrown completely off course.

168 A STITCH IN TIME

Don't waste time re-doing jobs you've rushed through and therefore done badly. Take a little extra time to do a proper job and you'll save time in the long run.

169 TURN OFF THE TV

If you're the sort of person who just can't find time to do anything in the evening, turning the TV off for an hour each evening will give you 365 hours (equivalent to 9 weeks) of extra time to achieve something.

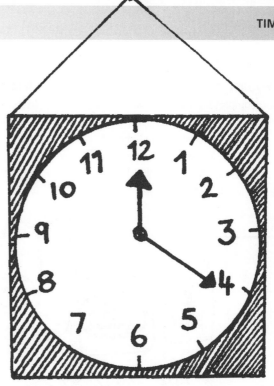

170 KEEP IT RELEVANT

Studies have shown that people who keep in mind the 'value' of their job are generally more satisfied. For instance, if you have to work overtime for a few weeks, remind yourself that the extra money will allow you to buy that treat you've wanted.

171 FREE YOUR TIME

People who feel really pressed for time often misuse it. Write a log of how much time you spend surfing the web, watching TV and dawdling in a week, then work out how you could have put it to more constructive use.

172 TREAT YOURSELF

When you complete a task or finish something as planned, give yourself a little treat. It could be something small like 20 minutes' rest with a magazine or something big like an evening out. This will help train your brain to want to finish tasks.

173 TAKE 24

Try to make sure that each week you have at least 24 hours when you don't think about work. Use it to see friends, get out of the house, spend time with your family and other things you enjoy. It will help you work better the following week.

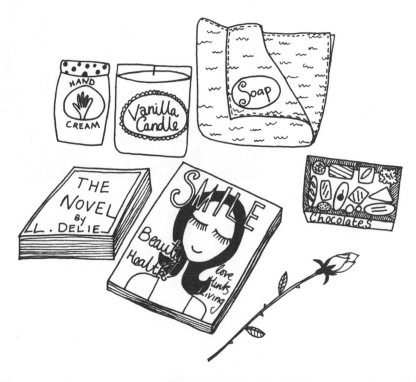

174 POP ON THE PASTA

For people with busy lives, pasta is a great choice for meals as it provides a slow-release source of energy to get you through the day. It's also really easy to make. Make it even easier by freezing some of your favourite pasta sauces for an instant meal. Throw in some in-season vegetables and you have a healthy meal.

175 BREAK UP BIG TASKS

If you find large tasks intimidating and overwhelming, split them into smaller tasks and do a little at a time. For instance, putting a year's worth of photos in albums might seem daunting, but not if you take a few at a time and spread it over several weeks.

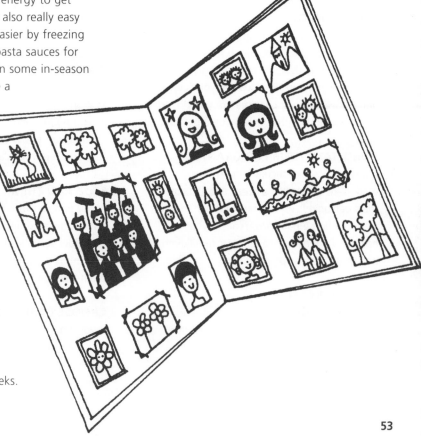

managing your lifestyle

176 TAKE CONTROL

Feeling powerless is a major cause of stress and it's the choices you make that determine whether you're running your life or it's running you. Even where you feel you don't have choices, chances are you do, so make decisions rather than avoiding them.

177 DON'T TAKE THEM FOR GRANTED

Many people – particularly men – who work hard and achieve great things take their personal lives and family for granted. To boost home harmony, realize what you have and remember to let your family know how much you appreciate them.

178 BE CHOOSY

Everything in your life is not equal, and it's important to see it that way. Re-evaluate the amount of time you spend on tasks and with people, according to how important they are to you.

179 KNOW YOUR LIMITS

Don't be drawn into spending longer and longer at work to get your jobs done. Talk to your boss or line manager about the number of extra hours they can reasonably expect of you and stick to your limits.

180 WRITE A REVIEW

Every six months or so, review your priorities at work. If your job is not working as well as you had hoped, look at what needs to be changed and how you can make it work so that you feel your career is on track.

181 STOP AND THINK

Many people work hard because they find it difficult to stop and relax, or are frightened to. Allow some space into your life where nothing is planned to give your body and brain the chance to unwind.

182 CHOOSE CAREFULLY

If you find work takes over your life and it's all about income, think about changing careers for one you find more fulfilling; that way, it won't just be about money.

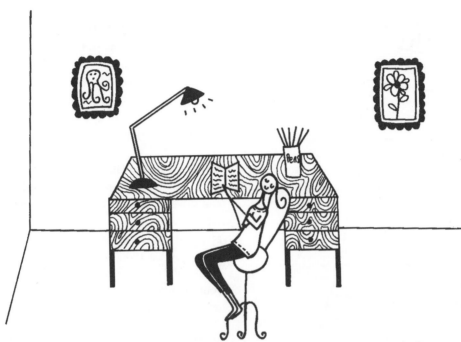

183 MAKE MORE TIME

If you're miserable at work, accept the fact that you need to give more time to yourself and your family in order to be happy. Then draw up your plan on paper so you can see for yourself which areas you need to give more attention to.

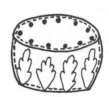

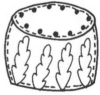

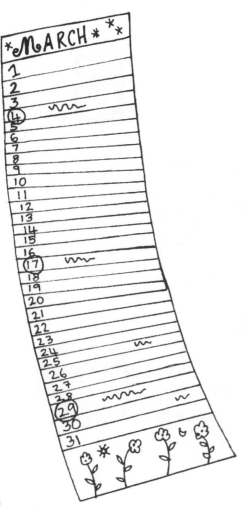

184 SET AN EARLY DEADLINE

If you're the sort of person who only works well when deadlines are near, use tricks to help organize your working life. For instance, set your deadline a few days before the real one to give you a cushion in case anything goes wrong.

185 GET A LIFE BALANCE

Keep your lifestyle expectations realistic, and strive for a balance of being happy at work and home. For instance, you may be prepared to sacrifice expensive holidays for fewer hours at work so that you can attend classes and learn a new skill. Deciding what your priorities are will help you make decisions more easily.

186 HOME PRIORITY

Some people think work is more important than home life, but most people who overwork have simply fallen into the habit of being that way. Putting the priority back on your home life could help you make decisions that make you feel happier both at home and at work.

187 DON'T OVERCOMPENSATE

If you're working because you feel high achievement makes you a better person, think again about your self-esteem. Try to find things you could do in other areas of your life that would help you feel as good.

188 A PARTY OF ONE

Ensure you have at least one evening a week for yourself and your family, when you don't allow work to be thought of or mentioned, and you simply enjoy each other's company.

189 JUST SAY NO

If you find it difficult to say no at work, practise in the mirror or with friends or a partner. Get them to ask you the sort of question you would usually find it difficult to say no to and practise your response.

190 YOU'RE NUMBER ONE

Don't let your work become the most important thing in your life – make sure you are always number one in the decisions you make. Look after yourself and you'll end up happier and healthier.

191 GET A MANTRA

If you find yourself getting stressed and overwhelmed by work during the day, choose a phrase that reminds you to relax ('slow down, breathe better' or 'I can feel the space inside my head'). Then close your eyes and repeat the phrase to yourself when you feel stress levels rising.

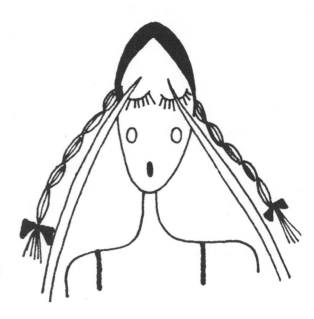

192 LEARN TO DELEGATE

You'll never be able to do everything on your own, so learn the art of delegation. That means trusting people to complete tasks on their own, not hovering over them and wasting both your time and theirs.

193 GET SOME PERSPECTIVE

It's all too easy to lose perspective when you're working too hard, but life is more rewarding when work and personal life are balanced. You'll be surprised at how acknowledging a problem can help you enact a beneficial change.

194 TAKE AN INVENTORY

Many people have regular reviews at work, and it's a valuable tool to help you address problems and aspirations. Give yourself a career review every six months and check everything is working towards your goals.

195 DON'T GIVE 140%

It's fine to give all of yourself to your job when you're doing it, but make a rule that evenings are to be work free.

healthy finances

196 OWN UP TO DEBT

If you're going to solve your financial problems with your partner, it's important you own up to debt and work together to solve problems. Don't be secretive about your spending habits. Make the time to work out budgets together.

197 SHARE THE WEALTH

If you're the wage earner, never use money as a weapon. The way people deal with money in a relationship says a lot about who has the power, the freedom and the control, so make sure you keep it as equal as possible.

198 BE A SPENDTHRIFT

A major cause of money worries is over-spending and increasing debt. For a month, don't allow yourself to buy anything that isn't absolutely essential. Be strict and at the end of that period, you'll be amazed at how little you've missed those things you thought were so important.

199 DO DIRECT

Choose direct debit for utility and credit card bills. You'll ensure you won't pay interest charges by missing dates and most companies offer discounts for direct debit payments.

200 GO ONLINE

Shop online for essentials and you'll find you can do it every two weeks rather than every week. You will save yourself time and money and remove the stress of carrying lots of stuff around a crowded supermarket and having to make on-the-spot decisions.

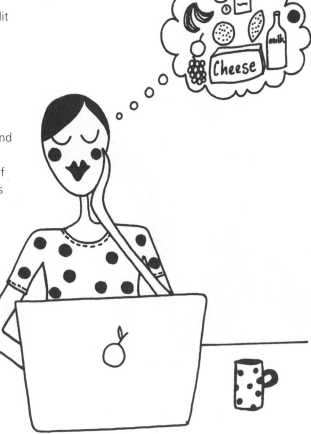

201 THINK AHEAD

Book travel and entertainment tickets in advance rather than a few days beforehand. Often, you'll find you get better deals and it will take the stress out of that last-minute booking. This is particularly true of travel to foreign destinations at peak times of the year.

202 BE VIGILANT

Check through your credit history carefully and if there's anything you think is strange, like a loan application you didn't make, you could be a victim of ID fraud. Get in touch with the lender immediately to make sure. Your credit report changes all the time, so it's important to check it regularly to make sure it's up to date and there are no mistakes or problems.

203 PRIORITIZE PAYMENTS

If you're worried about paying all your debts, don't just pay the one that shouts loudest. Work out which debts and expenses are your priorities – for instance, mortgage, rent, tax and utilities – and pay them first.

204 SHOP SMART

Try to buy things that aren't essential in sales or at discount outlets. Make it your aim never to pay full price for nonessential items and you'll get the feel-good boost of having bagged a bargain as well as saving yourself money.

205 SEPARATE YOUR FINANCES

When the financial credit check companies go through your report, they may also check the reports of people with whom you have had financial dealings in the past, like joint accounts or loans, which may impact your credit rating. If you are separated, make sure your finances are, too.

206 DON'T BE DISTRACTED

When it comes to choosing a bank account, don't be distracted by 'free gifts' and special offers which can often mask lower interest rates or higher fees. Choose the account that works for you best.

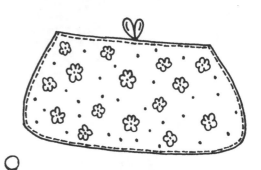

207 THINK AHEAD

Get a pension as soon as you can, which will help you reduce those worries about what will happen as you get older. The longer you save for, the less you will pay, so sooner is best.

208 THE REAL COSTS

Before you sign up for store cards, credit cards and loans, get out your calculator and work out exactly how much you will be paying back and make sure you'll be able to afford the repayments.

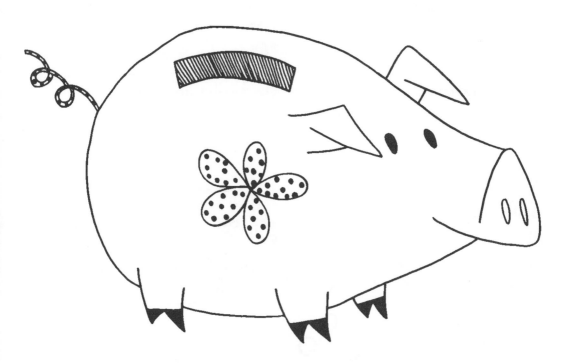

209 LET LENDERS KNOW

If you are struggling with repayments, don't hide your head in the sand. Many companies now have protocols in place to help people who are struggling, including freezing and reducing repayments.

210 OPEN YOUR BILLS

Always open your bills and bank statements and read through them, particularly if you are having money problems. Ignoring them won't make problems go away and you're best off knowing the whole picture.

211 TALK TO CREDITORS

If you need to stop some repayments, talk to your creditors first rather than just going ahead. If you explain your problems, they are likely to be more understanding.

212 DON'T ROB PETER TO PAY PAUL

Avoid falling into the trap of borrowing money or taking out a loan to pay off existing debt. This is likely to lead to many more problems in the long run and will mean you pay more interest.

213 MAKE CONTACT

If you find something in your credit check you disagree with, make sure you contact the relevant lender or authority in writing as soon as possible. Keeping a record of correspondence can help settle issues.

214 REGISTER TO VOTE

Money lenders use the electoral register (voter registration) to check that you are who you say you are and that you live at your address as a protection against fraud. Make sure your information is up to date.

215 REDUCE YOUR DEBTS

Instead of owing small amounts of money to lots of creditors, try to pay off a few entirely. Not only will this be easier to manage but it will look better on your credit score.

216 TELL THE TRUTH

Don't lie or bend the truth in any way on an application form for finances. It might seem like a small thing but it counts as fraud and could leave a permanent black mark on your credit rating.

finding your vocation

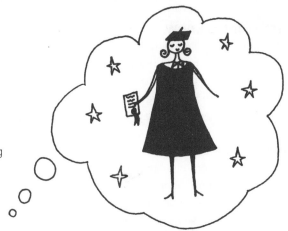

217 DO YOUR RESEARCH

Once you've decided on a vocation or career that you think is right for you, do some research to check there isn't anything that puts you off before you take the plunge. Look for things like salary ranges, educational requirements, working hours and conditions.

218 GET SOME VALUE

Working out what your values are is an important part of choosing the right career. There is no right or wrong when it comes to values, it's simply what you hold dear. Be honest with yourself.

219 THE REAL YOU

If you want to find a good career match you've got to know what makes you tick. Don't listen to what your friends and family think, because the only one who really knows what's in your heart is you.

220 MEASURE YOUR EXCITEMENT

A good gauge of what is likely to motivate you in a career is what keeps you awake and interested in general life. Make a list of things you're really into and try to think of a career that would combine them.

221 LOCATION LOCATION

If you're trying to choose the right career, think about where you'll work as well as the job. For instance, do you see yourself as an office person or more of an outdoors type? Do you like quiet or bustle?

222 WORK ON YOUR SKILLS

Having an interest in a certain career – or even a talent for it – doesn't count if you haven't got the skills to match. Volunteer, take classes and work on honing your skills to suit the job you want.

223 DON'T BE EMBARRASSED

If you have strange interests or interests that aren't the same as your family and friends, don't be pressured into doing what they do. Be honest with yourself about what you like and you'll be happier for it.

224 UNEARTH YOUR TALENT

Talent is important because it makes us feel good about ourselves. Chances are, you'll probably like the things you're good at. If you don't know what your talents are, ask your nearest and dearest for their thoughts.

225 TAKE A TEST DRIVE

If you're thinking of starting a career path or changing careers, why not give it a test drive first? Volunteer or job shadow so you can see what the job is really like.

226 BE OPEN-MINDED

When it comes to choosing a career, it isn't just about how well you perform academically. Consider how you relate to others – are you a born leader, well organized or good at putting people at ease? These too are important things to consider.

227 CHOOSE THE JOB FOR YOU

Your work is part of your life, not your whole life, but chances are you spend more time at your place of work than at your home. Make sure you choose a job that works for you rather than being pushed into something you don't like.

228 FOLLOW TRENDS

If you want to find the right career, it's important to have your finger on the pulse when it comes to new trends and how they alter the jobs on offer in the workplace. This will help you plan a career being mindful of changing technology. Read the jobs pages in the newspapers and talk to other people about what's happening.

work it out

229 WALK IT OUT

If possible, try to work near where you live. Studies have shown that people whose home-to-work journeys are less than half an hour are significantly less stressed, especially if they can walk to work.

230 BRING YOUR FAMILY TO WORK

It has been proven that people who feel relaxed at their desks are more productive. Within reason, make your work environment more appealing with family photos, plants or other decorations. Don't let paperwork build up around you. Clear the clutter and put things into containers.

231 SET PRIORITIES

Don't let small, insignificant tasks get in the way of big ones. If you have trouble prioritizing, try writing lists in a colour system, with red for 'essential', black for 'required' and blue for 'optional', and concentrate on red first to make sure you don't lose track of what's important.

232 GET GOSSIPING

Don't spend your well-earned tea break talking or thinking about work – your brain will function much better on your return if you give it a complete rest, and studies have shown that gossiping is good for productivity!

233 GO PUBLIC

Make sure you forward plan when it comes to your job so you aren't surprised by sudden increases in workload. Think ahead and talk to someone who can help beforehand if you think you're going to struggle rather than waiting until it's all too much.

234 MAKE ONE JOURNEY

Try to work out your journey to work so you rely on one mode of transport only. Changing from car to train to bus is the most stressful part of commuting.

235 REAP THE REWARD

Whether it's a home or work project, you'll benefit from setting targets. Divide your project into long- and short-term goals and give yourself a treat whenever you reach one.

236 FANTASTIC FOLIAGE

One of the best ways to help you feel healthier and happier at work, especially if you find yourself surrounded by electrical equipment, is to invest in a few plants. They will help absorb radioactive waves, remove toxic pollutants from the atmosphere and will help you feel calmer too. Research has shown that workers are more productive if there are plants in their offices. Buy one for your desk: peace lilies, areca palms, Boston ferns and dracaenas are all good choices.

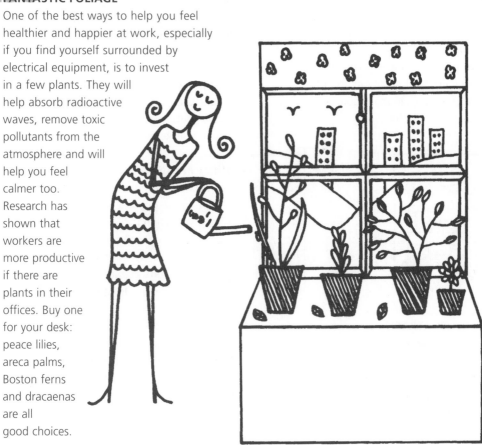

237 COOK UP A STORM

Food is really important to maintain brainpower. If you've got a big project coming up at work and are likely to be too tired to cook in the evening, make up a few batches of nutritious food for the freezer so you can make sure your brain stays in tiptop form.

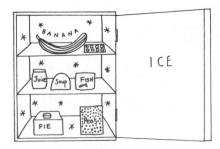

238 CUT THE NEGATIVITY

For a whole week, don't allow yourself to say anything negative about anyone else at work. Stopping yourself will make you realize how negative you can be and how much it affects you. Try to find positive things to say about your co-workers.

office angels

239 KNOW YOUR ENERGY

Take a few days thinking about what is your most productive time of day and try to organize your time around them. For instance, if you have a natural dip at 4 pm, maybe that's a good time to do tasks that require a little less brainpower.

240 DON'T PROCRASTINATE

Open your post immediately rather than leaving it in unopened piles. Throw away or recycle anything you don't need to keep and try to file everything else straight away, keeping out only what you need to deal with. Aim to look at each piece of paper only once and don't let it pile up.

241 AN EARLY BIRD

If you often find yourself rushed and flustered when you get to the office, start getting up 15 minutes earlier. The extra time will give you a chance to read through your work notes for the day so that you can start the day feeling well prepared.

242 GIVE YOURSELF A BREAK

Did you know that 91 million working days a year are lost to mental ill-health in the UK and in the USA 200 million working days are lost annually? Working till you drop isn't going to do anyone any favours in the long run, so make sure you give yourself regular breaks to stay on top of things.

243 MAKE A LIST

Before you leave work at night, make a fresh list for the next day and stick it on your screen or desktop or leave it open on your desk. It will stop you wasting time the next day and help your head stay clear in the evening.

244 BE REALISTIC

If you're commuting in the winter, make sure you allow more time as many accidents are caused by people rushing in inclement weather. Planning journeys in advance will make you less stressed.

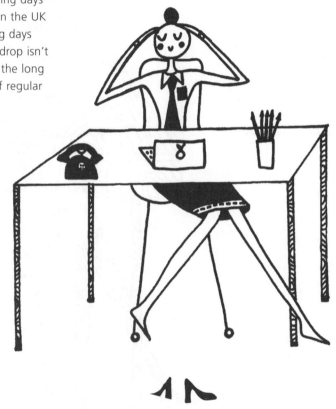

245 A GOOD POSITION

Make sure your chair is comfortable
and your lower back is supported,
and that you're not too far from
your keyboard. Nothing should
feel strained or stretched,
especially if you stay in the
same position for a while.

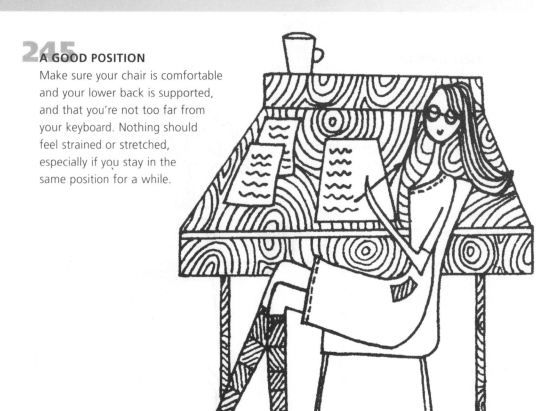

246 CLEAN IT UP

Invest 5 minutes of time in cleaning up your desk before you leave the office – arriving to a clutter-free desk in the morning will help you start the day on the right note.

247 TELL THE TIME

Make sure you have a clock on your desk or prominently displayed on your computer. That way, you'll be able to monitor how long it takes you to do things so time doesn't run away with you.

248 GET ELECTRONIC

Buy an electronic organizer, or use your phone or BlackBerry, to serve as your diary, address book and calendar. Using it to remember things like birthdays as well as meetings will free up brain space for more efficient working.

249 CREATE A SYSTEM

Spend a few hours making sure your filing system is clear and concise and that it works for you. It's stressful not to be able to find essential items when you need them.

250 COMMUNICATE WITH STAFF

If you're a manager, don't get so bogged down in trying to assign tasks that you forget to ask your workers what they want – research has shown that people work best if they enjoy their role, so keep in the loop.

251 HOLD A MEETING

When there are big decisions to be made, it's always best to meet face to face (or at least by video link if a face-to-face meeting isn't possible) because it's human nature to want to see reactions.

252 CHOOSE A BAD JOB

Work through your to do list sensibly – don't choose all the jobs you like first and leave the bad jobs till last. Instead, try to alternate an enjoyable job with one you don't feel like doing.

253 GET MOBILE

Instead of being stuck in the office, buy a laptop so you can move your office with you and maximize flexibility – get one with a built-in fax facility.

254 TELEPHONE TENNIS

Return a call once, leaving a message and telling the person when you are available. Make sure you're available when you say you will be and you'll avoid wasting time to-ing and fro-ing with answer messages.

255 EAT LIGHT

At lunchtime, make sure you don't overeat and try to avoid too much caffeine and alcohol which might cause a dip in energy in the afternoon. Keep lunch light and energizing with salads, fruit and protein.

256 MULTITASK

Jobs that aren't too critical and don't require 140% concentration can be joined together to save time; for instance, deleting junk emails or organizing papers while talking on the phone.

257 KEEP IT BRIEF

Try to keep work phone calls brief and to the point. Spend a minute deciding what you want to say beforehand and try not to be distracted.

258 SET A STANDARD

To save time when you're sending emails or letters, try to create standard templates you can use so you don't have to worry about starting afresh each time. This will help you free up more office time for other tasks.

259 GET OUT AND ABOUT

Your office will work more efficiently if everyone has a lunch break. Try to encourage everyone to go out for at least a 10 or 15 minute break to perk them up and keep them going for the rest of the day.

260 BE PREPARED

If possible, try to set out your clothes the night before so you don't rush in the morning. If you take a packed lunch to work, make sure it's already prepared so you can get out of the door quickly.

261 SOUND OF SILENCE

In laboratory experiments, it has been shown that mice who were played irritating noises found it harder to concentrate. Make sure your office is free of audible irritations.

262 FILE IT AWAY

Make a scheduled time to do your filing every day so papers don't get on top of you. It's an easy job, so right after your lunch break or later in the afternoon is usually a good time to choose.

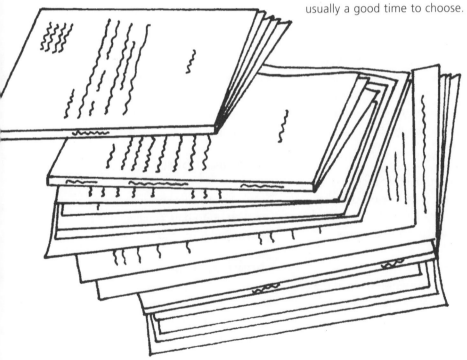

263 PAIN BEFORE PLEASURE

It might be tempting to do all the enjoyable things in your life first, but studies show you'll actually enjoy your leisure time more if you feel you've achieved something beforehand – so work now, play later.

264 GET COMPETITIVE

To help keep you all motivated and if you have co-workers who are interested, get them involved in deadline competitions for tasks or see who delivers the best quality product or service within the time.

265 CLEAN OUT

Make it a rule to get together every month in the office to clear it of unwanted papers and accumulated junk. Put on some music and go through everything to declutter.

266 ASK FOR QUIET

If certain colleagues cause disruption in the office, why not instigate a 'quiet' period every day or ask for a 'red flag' system where you can ask for calm if you've got important work or preparation to do.

267 CLUB THINGS TOGETHER

If your job can be split into different compartments like making sales calls, sending emails, creative thinking time etc, try to lump them together into separate time blocks so you can work more efficiently.

268 GIVE PRAISE

Every time someone does something on time at work or at home, make sure you show your appreciation. Workers will be prepared to go that extra mile if they feel their efforts are appreciated.

269 STAY UP-TO-DATE

If you work from home or have a small office, make sure you concentrate on getting up-to-date equipment like integrated faxes and scanners.

270 DON'T MEET UP

Avoid unnecessary meetings, which can be a big drain on your precious time. If something can be resolved without a meeting, do so, but stick strictly to agendas if you do meet up.

271 KEEP WORK SEPARATE

If possible, try not to take work home
with you and if you must, then try to limit
it to one or two pre-planned nights a week.
Similarly, make it a rule if at all possible,
not to take your home life into the office.
Keep phone calls to lunchbreaks if there are
things you need to sort out.

272 BE AN ENERGIZER

Many of us like to have a good moan,
but did you know that lack of energy
and motivation is contagious? If you feel
energetic, you'll help the people around you
feel energetic, too, which makes everyone
happier. Make an effort to be positive
around your workmates for a week and
see the difference.

273 TRACK YOUR TIME

Keep a diary detailing what you do for a
week and at the end of the week tot up
the amount of time you spent on various
different tasks. Use it to plan your own
time or talk to your manager about
changing things if necessary.

274 THINK ABOUT IT

If someone asks you to take on more
responsibility at work, don't say yes
immediately just because you feel flattered.
Ask for time to think about it and really
stop and evaluate what it would mean to
your time management. Will it make your
job more stressful and can you really
manage to fit it in?

275 GET CALLER DISPLAY

Buying a caller display unit is a great way
to cut down on phone interruptions
because you can see who's calling before
you pick up the phone. You can then make
a decision about whether to pick it up or
leave it to go to answerphone.

276 IGNORE THE PHONE

It's all to easy to pick up the phone the
instant it rings but if you find you are
constantly being interrupted by calls, try
to have a time devoted to the telephone
and a period during the day when you
turn it off or switch it to answerphone
and concentrate on your other jobs.

homeworking

277 WORK BETTER HOURS

People who work from home are up to 20% more efficient than their office-based colleagues, probably due to the 'social distraction' factor. If you are on a contract or using flexitime to work at home, ask your bosses if your working day can reflect this with longer breaks or shorter hours.

278 A TELECOMMUTER

If you find getting to work is taking up too much of your day, see if you can negotiate working from home a few days a week, then use the time you would have spent travelling to exercise, relax or do something else that makes you feel good.

279 LOOK AWAY

People who work from home are much less likely to take breaks and look after themselves. Make sure you give your eyes a break from the screen every 15 minutes or so for at least a minute and use it as thinking time.

280 EAT OUT

It's often tempting to eat lunch in the office if you're working from home, but try to give yourself at least one proper break during the day. Allocate half an hour and try to eat lunch in another room, or even go out for lunch.

281 GET A LINE

To avoid unnecessary disturbances, get a separate business telephone line for when you're working from home and don't give the number to family and friends.

282 BE SELECTIVE

Joining email groups and lists can be tempting, but make sure you police their activity – some groups generate a large number of emails that could be distracting if you're trying to work.

283 SET A RECORD

It's fine to watch TV during break times if you're working from home, but don't let it set your timetables. If there are programmes you want to watch, record them so your work won't suffer.

284 TAKE A BREAK

Don't fall into the trap of spending the whole day inside if you're working from home. If the weather's nice, hand-deliver a package, take a letter to the post office, or go for a walk.

285 MAKE THE CALL

It's fine to allow yourself a non-work-related phone call during your day working at home; just make sure you keep it within a specified time and don't let it become a distraction.

286 DO A CHECK

Set specific times when you will check your emails rather than checking them constantly throughout the day. Four times a day should be enough to keep you informed but undistracted. If you're expecting important emails, make sure colleagues know to call you so that you don't miss a deadline.

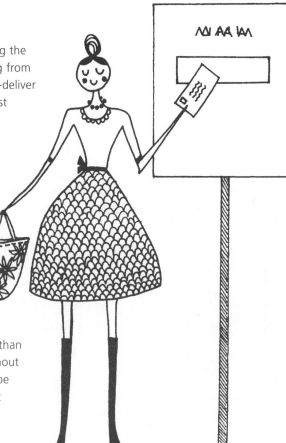

287 TURN OFF THE TV

While having the TV on in the background may help reduce feelings of isolation, it can be very distracting. Radio is a better option, or music played through your computer. Classical music is less distracting and stress relieving than other forms of music – Mozart is apparently the composer most likely to make you feel happy!

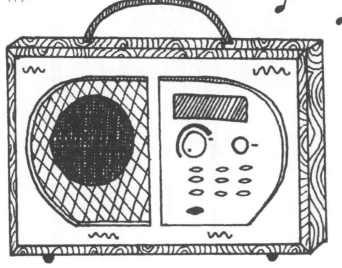

288 MEET UP

Schedule a meeting or lunch with co-workers to get yourself out of your home office at lunchtime. It will help you catch up on what's happening in the office as well as give you a break from your surroundings.

289 GET A REVIEW

Just because you work from home, don't lose out on the regular reviews and progress reports you are entitled to if you work in an office. Schedule a regular timeslot with your line manager to keep you in the loop.

290 WORK SPACE ONLY

Make sure you have a separate area used only for working, so you can leave paperwork around without the dog dribbling on it and you are still able to walk away at the end of the day and switch off.

291 GET A SEPARATE ACCOUNT

Email is great for keeping in touch, but it can be a distraction. Think about setting up different accounts for work and leisure, and be strict about using them.

292 DON'T BE DISTRACTED

One of the biggest problems for people working in offices is the distractions they deal with each day, but working from home can be difficult too – try to set a clear space for working in and make sure your family know the boundaries of your time.

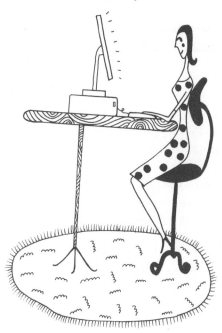

293 SAY NO TO FRIENDS

Ironically, it's often not colleagues who cause a problem when you're working from home, but family and friends who think if you're not in the office it's a day off. Let them know you're not available during working hours.

294 CUT-OFF HOUR

Just because you are a home or remote worker, it doesn't mean you have to become a prisoner of your work. Make sure you stick to your working hours and don't be tempted to carry on into the evening on a regular basis.

295 GET A FILTER

Set up filters in your email program to sort and keep track of email (this is particularly important if you can't have separate work and leisure accounts). This way, you'll be more able to separate work and home life.

296 DO SOME CHORES

If you work from home, set yourself break times and use those times to achieve something in the house – that way, you'll be less likely to be distracted when your break ends. Try a load of laundry or washing up. And don't forget lunch.

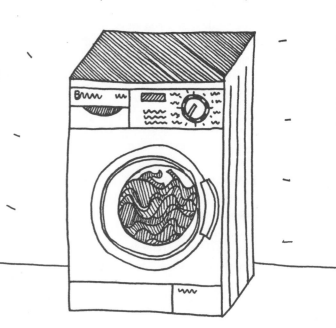

back to work

287 BACK TO WORK

Going back to work after a baby is a big decision. Make sure you've weighed up the pros and cons by writing a list and really thinking about what's best for your family. Some mothers would be miserable without the extra money or adult time, but others would feel guilty or resent the intrusion of work into family life.

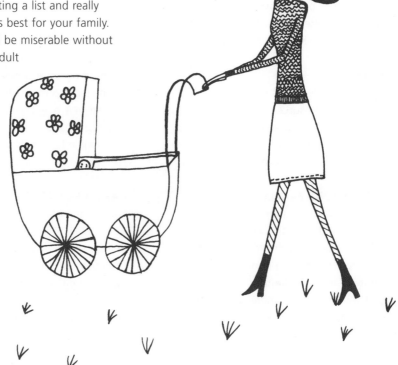

298 SHARE THE LOAD

Before you decide to go back to work, make an inventory of your family life and think of all the ways you could make it work. For instance, some families find that both parents working part-time works better than one full-time and one at home with the children.

299 GET REAL

Make your expectations realistic so you allow yourself to succeed. It's impossible to be perfect in every area of life so allow for some failure and for some things to not be done as well as you'd like.

300 INVOLVE YOUR FAMILY

Discuss any changes that are due to take place with your family when you sit down together at mealtimes. Let them be involved in deciding how everyone can contribute to make the transition easier. Apart from child care, there are household tasks to reassign.

301 ASK FOR ADVICE

If you're going back to work after having children, involve your employer in making the transition easier – do they have flexible hours, courses on time management or subsidized child care which could help you?

302 CHANGE CAREER

Going back to work after having children doesn't necessarily mean going back to the same job. Don't be afraid to choose a career that is less demanding on time and nerves if it seems like the best decision for the whole family. Why not visit a career advisor to help you decide?

303 ASK A FRIEND

Rather than taking the leap back to work alone, talk to your friends and family who have already made that transition for ideas on how they coped and any possible pitfalls they encountered. Take advantage of hindsight and learn from other people's mistakes.

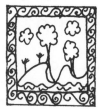

304 PLAN A REST

When you plan out your day do not forget
to include rest and recreation time for
yourself, and don't treat it as an indulgence.
Relaxed, rested people are far better able
to cope with life's ups and downs and
come out on top.

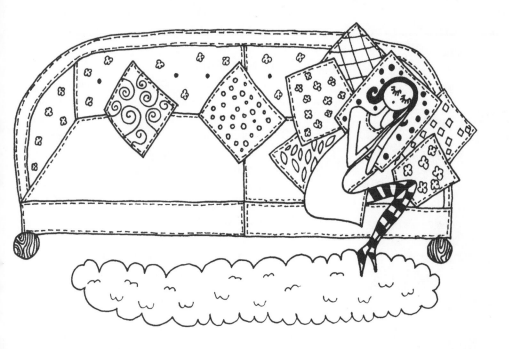

supplements & diet

305 FEEL GOOD WITH FOLATE

The supplement folate is thought to help reduce mental disorders and a lack of it is linked to increased rates of depression, possibly due to a reduction in the body's ability to make serotonin.

306 NICE NIACIN

Niacin has been shown to be effective at improving circulation, reducing cholesterol and helping prevent diabetes, osteoarthritis and cataracts, but supplements can cause side effects. If you suffer these, eat protein foods instead, from which the body can create its own niacin.

307 CHOOSE SEEDS

Lots of people take flaxseed oil to help boost their levels of healthy cholesterols and triglycerides, but the ground-up seeds are an even better choice as they also contain anti-viral lignans, which can boost immunity.

308 GET FISHY

Taking a daily supplement of omega-3 oils is a great choice for overall health as they have been linked not only to increased physical and mental performance but also to a reduction in depression.

309 READ A MAG

Not only can magnesium help palpitations, muscle cramps and menopausal symptoms, some studies have shown that it can help reduce blood pressure as well, so make sure you're getting enough in a supplement form or from green leafy vegetables such as spinach, figs, aubergines (eggplants), sweetcorn, seeds and raisins.

310 BE A KAVAMAN

Kava kava is a herb often used to reduce anxiety but be careful not to take too much as it has been associated with liver damage. See your doctor if you want to take it regularly for more than a few weeks and don't take it without seeking advice if you're on any other medication, are pregnant, breastfeeding or have Parkinson's disease.

311 CUT CRAMPS

Vitamin B6 is thought to reduce muscle cramps, stiffness of the hands, nausea, depression and dry skin and it is an excellent natural diuretic, which means it boosts fluid drainage.

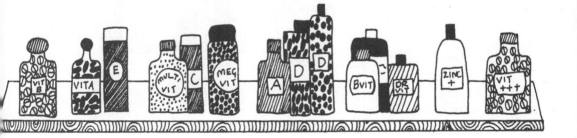

312 SELECT SELENIUM

Selenium is a trace mineral thought to be excellent for heart health and it also facilitates the absorption of vitamin E, but try not to take selenium at the same time as vitamin C, which may block its effects.

313 A CO-WORKER

Co-enzyme Q10 is said to be an antioxidant that can improve energy utilization and boost heart health. Levels start to decrease from the age of about 35, so it's worth starting to boost levels then.

314 BE CHASTE

Chaste tree berry extract is a source of natural phyto-oestrogens and can be useful to women suffering symptoms of PMS or menopause by helping the body to regulate fluctuating hormone levels.

315 TOP UP TAURINE

Taurine is an amino acid that is a potent antitoxin and antioxidant and is vital for the liver and immune system as well as being a great choice for reducing anxiety and boosting heart health. Get it from meat (especially red meat) or supplements.

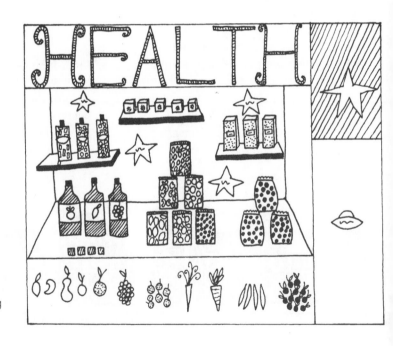

316 DO IT WITH DHEA

A hormone naturally produced by the body, high levels of DHEA are linked to longer life, lower production of fat cells and an increase in the body's ability to utilize energy and burn fat, as well as reducing the risk of cancer.

317 TRY TYROSINE

The nonessential amino acid tyrosine has been found to play a role in controlling depression and can also help speed up the metabolism and treat conditions characterized by chronic fatigue. Tyrosine aids in the production of melanin (pigment of the skin and hair) and boosts the function of the adrenal, thyroid and pituitary glands.

318 GET HEALTHY MUSCLES

If your muscles are tired and fatigued a lot of the time, make sure you're getting enough of the amino acid L-carnitine, which is essential for muscle function. It is a great choice for weight maintenance as well as heart health.

319 BORON FOR BONES

A lack of the trace mineral boron is thought to be linked to decreased bone and joint function. If you're taking a multivitamin designed for joints, make sure it contains boron.

320 HAVE A GOOD EVENING

Evening primrose oil has been shown to help reduce the symptoms of PMS and menopause and is excellent for hot flushes, breast tenderness and fluid retention as well as helping alleviate depression.

321 GO FOR GINKGO

Ginkgo biloba is often taken for its ability to improve memory, but it can also be helpful in alleviating depression and enhancing your capacity to relax. Get advice from your doctor if you're using anticoagulants.

322 LOOK FOR LECITHIN

Soy lecithin is often found in processed foods as it is a natural emulsifier, but taking the substance (as granules) could help your body reduce circulating fats.

323 VOTE FOR VALERIAN

Often used as a natural sleep aid because of its relaxation effects, valerian root can also be used to help treat anxiety. Choose the capsule form if you don't like the (very pungent) smell of the natural root.

324 CHOOSE COHOSH

Black cohosh is a natural hormone precursor which is thought to be the ultimate women's herb as it enhances the reproductive system and helps reduce the effects of menopause and PMS, as well as lowering blood pressure.

325 Z IS FOR ZINC

Zinc is a great stressbuster so make sure you're either taking a supplement or eating zinc-rich foods like oysters, wholewheat, popcorn, muesli, eggs, cheese, nuts and seeds, especially at times of stress.

326 B HEALTHY

Take a look in the mirror and note any unusual differences. For example, if you are suffering from problem, tired skin, it could well be due to a lack of B vitamins. Take a B-complex or make sure you eat enough yogurt, liver, dates, beans and avocado.

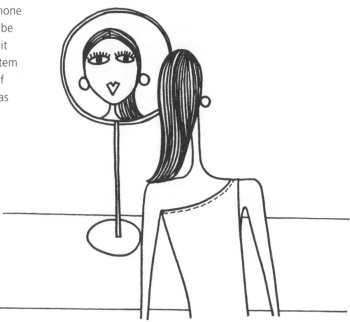

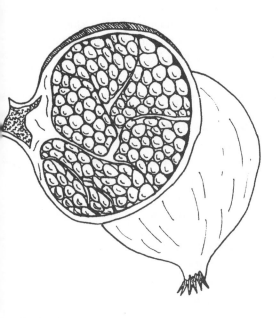

natural remedies

328 YOUR FIVE-A-DAY

To help keep your body in tiptop form, aim to eat at least five portions of fruit and vegetables daily, preferably seven to eight portions. A portion is about 80 g (3 oz), which is one apple, two plums, three dried apricots or half a cup of chopped vegetables, beans or pulses.

329 BE A CURRANT BUN

Blackcurrant is a great choice for boosting health and helping your body fight infection as it contains high levels of linoleic acid, linked to immunity as well as reducing breast tenderness. Eat berries or sip a natural tea for best effects.

327 C THE DIFFERENCE

In order to help your body stay well during stressful periods, you need to make sure your vitamin C levels stay high by taking a supplement or eating fruit and vegetables such as citrus, strawberries, pomegranates, kiwi, cabbage and broccoli.

330 HEAL A HEADACHE

One of the best natural remedies for headaches is feverfew, which is thought to dilate peripheral blood vessels, helping migraines, arthritis and allergies. It can interfere with blood clotting, though, so seek medical advice before taking.

331 HEAL WITH OIL

St John's wort isn't just a good herb to take for depression. If made into an oil (make your own by putting the leaves in oil in an airtight container and leaving in the sun for several days), it can be used to treat rashes and insect bites and stings.

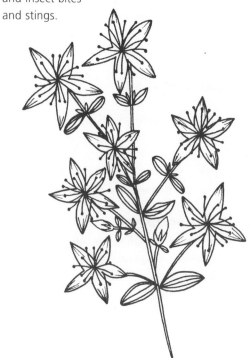

332 LICK STRESS AWAY

Liquorice is a great choice for reducing chronic stress, but it should be avoided if you also have high blood pressure. The most common formulation is a tincture or tea of liquorice root.

333 HAVE SOME HAWTHORN

Hawthorn dilates blood vessels and improves circulation as well as being thought to help keep your brain alert, but it's important to seek medical advice before taking it as it could interfere with other drugs.

334 CHOOSE CHAMOMILE

Chamomile is probably the most popular herb tea, known for its calming effects, but did you know it also helps protect against colds, flu, diarrhoea, menstrual cramping and drug withdrawal?

335 CRUSH A CRANBERRY

If you have urinary tract infections, inflammation or other problems, drink cranberry juice or use the berries raw in foods to help the urinary system heal itself.

336 THE GOOD AND BAD OF GINSENG

Ginseng is supposed to slow ageing, increase mental and physical capacity, aid sexual performance and boost immunity, but it does have the potential to elevate blood pressure, especially in those predisposed to hypertension. In addition, ginseng can increase sugar levels, which can be dangerous to diabetics, so take with caution and seek advice.

337 MAKE-AWAY NOT TAKE-AWAY

If you love your take-away food but want to be healthier, try making your own versions at home. Homemade pizzas, Chinese and curries are much lower in fat and salt and generally healthier than restaurant- or shop-bought options.

338 THE WHOLE STORY

Instead of processed foods and white flour products, choose wholemeal bread, brown rice, wholewheat pasta, porridge and potatoes with their skins on. These are higher in fibre and help your digestive system work effectively.

339 SIP A QUAI TEA

If you're suffering the ill effects of PMS or menopause, brewing up a tea of dong quai (which is related to the angelica family of plants) can help by regulating oestrogen use.

340 BE LEAN

Instead of fatty red meats every night, try to opt for lean meats like chicken, turkey, game or fish several times a week. This will help give you the protein energy boost you need without any of the extra fat, which can make you feel sluggish and less healthy in the long term.

341 RESCUE YOURSELF

Keep a vial of Bach flower Rescue Remedy with you at all times and put a few drops under your tongue to help you regain your calm if you feel angry, emotional, anxious or nervous.

342 HEALTHY FATS

Instead of choosing butter, lard or other meat and dairy fats, choose oils that won't raise cholesterol like extra-virgin olive, cold-pressed walnut, avocado or safflower oils.

343 DITCH THE SUGAR

Not only can sugar affect your moods, making you feel low, it also uses up essential stress-busting vitamins like the B complex. Replace with honey, maple syrup, puréed fruit, dates or raisins.

detoxing

344 DON'T BE A FAKE

Try to avoid 'fake' foods like artificial sweeteners, colouring, flavouring and preservatives. Aim to consume as many of your foods in their natural state as you can. Organic produce is free from pesticides and additives and it is also cultivated according to principles that enhance the beneficial vitamins and minerals they contain.

345 FLUSH YOUR LIVER

Squeeze the juice of a grapefruit and a lemon into a glass and dilute with filtered water, then add the juice of one clove of garlic, a knob of fresh ginger and a touch of extra-virgin olive oil. Stir and sip slowly for a liver-cleansing detox drink.

346 DETOX THROUGH YOUR DIET

If you're feeling sluggish – particularly if you've been eating out and drinking and your liver is suffering – choose a diet rich in foods that cleanse the liver and eliminate toxins, such as celery, spinach, banana, onion, garlic, grapefruit and pear.

347 CHEW THE FAT

Make sure you chew your food thoroughly to aid digestion – unchewed food can accumulate in the bowel and cause sluggishness, so chewing properly and not rushing your meal is essential.

348 START WITH LEMON

At the beginning of each day, kickstart your kidneys and other organs with a glass of warm water and freshly squeezed lemon juice. Add a little honey for sweetness.

349 SIP IT UP

Make sure every meal is accompanied with a glass of filtered water and sip regularly as you eat to help food pass easily through your system. This is especially important if you're also drinking alcohol with a meal.

350 EAT LITTLE AND OFTEN

To help the body detox, it's better to eat little and often, which also keeps your metabolism ticking over. Eating three large meals overloads the digestive system.

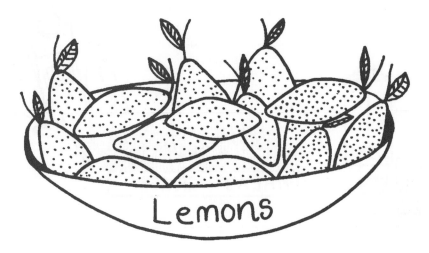

Lemons

351 CUT THE WHEAT

A good starting point for detoxing is to cut out wheat, including bread, cakes and pasta. Instead opt for bread and foods made from oats, rice, rye and spelt flour.

352 EARLY TO BED

Your body does its healing at night, so while you're undertaking a detox aim to be in bed early to give it lots of time to heal from the inside out. Half past ten is a good time as it allows for a long refreshing sleep, no matter what time you have to get up.

353 AVOID TRANS FATS

Don't eat foods containing hydrogenated fats or trans fats, which have been shown to be dangerous because they affect heart health and could be carcinogenic.

354 SIP SPIRULINA

Try to include one portion per day of detox foods like spirulina, alfalfa sprouts or wheatgrass in your diet. These boost your intake of nutrients, which can help the detoxification process.

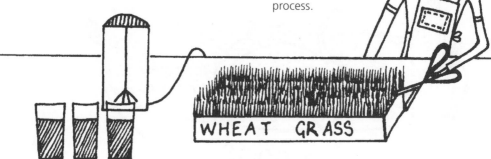

WHEAT GRASS

355 DROP THE DAIRY

Cut out most of your dairy intake, including milk, cheese, ice cream and cream. Small amounts of butter and eggs are fine, but try replacing milk with soya, rice or oat milk products instead.

356 AVOID BACON AND HAM

Instead of choosing bacon and ham, which contain lots of salt, go for fresher meats like chicken and beef, which are unpreserved. That way, you can be sure you're making a healthy choice.

357 TAKE A PILL

If you're doing a detox, boost your body's natural detox capabilities with supplements. Specialist detox supplements are the ideal choice for short-term use, and psyllium husks can help remove toxins.

358 BRUSH UP

You can boost your natural removal of toxins by using a body brush to encourage your circulation, which in turn helps aid lymphatic drainage. Always brush towards the heart.

keeping healthy

359 EAT RIGHT

A balanced diet can help you reduce stress by keeping blood sugar levels constant and avoiding the peaks and troughs which can lead to mood swings.

360 KEEP YOUR MEDICATION WITH YOU

When you go away, make sure you take any essential medication and keep a spare prescription with you in case you lose your drugs. That way, you'll be able to relax better.

361 REDUCE PAIN

Some foods are naturally thought to have pain-relieving properties so are great choices if you want to control pain without drugs. Ginger and turmeric are particularly effective for chronic pain.

362 ASK A QUESTION

When you're suffering a chronic condition such as arthritis, the pain can be with you much of the time. Write down questions and queries about your condition as they occur to you and take the list to your doctor during your next visit so they don't slip your mind.

363 MAKE EXERCISE FUN

If you find exercise boring, dull or really hard work, try enrolling in a form of activity that will make it more fun and sociable. Dancing, walking with groups, aqua classes and tai chi are all good choices.

364 REDUCE INFLAMMATION

Foods that are thought to reduce inflammation include olives, onions, grapes, raisins and green tea so try to include these in your diet if you have an inflammatory condition like arthritis.

365 THINK SPIRITUALLY

Nobody quite knows why, but research shows that people who have spiritual belief or who pray regularly generally feel better both emotionally and physically than people who don't, so embrace a higher power for greater wellbeing.

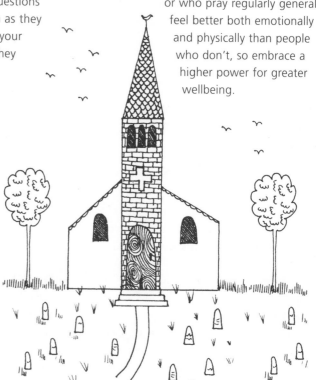

366 SEE A THERAPIST

If you are worried that your diet might be exacerbating a chronic condition such as arthritis or eczema, seek help from a qualified nutritional therapist who will be able to help you pinpoint trigger foods.

367 BUILD AN UNDERSTANDING

Knowing your disease will help you manage it, so don't just accept what you know about your condition – try to learn something new about it as the knowledge base is likely to be changing all the time. Research your condition on the internet but make sure the information sources are reputable and professional. You can also find details of support groups.

368 TAKE A STEP

Previously, experts believed 10,600 steps a day was enough to control weight, but an international study has just established that women up to the age of 40 and men up to 50 need 12,600 steps a day to help shift that midriff. Invest in a pedometer to make sure you're hitting your target.

teeth & gums

369 VISIT YOUR DENTIST

Make sure you see your dentist every six months so they can make sure your teeth and gums are healthy. Don't be afraid to ask questions and make sure you alert them to any problems you've been having. If they don't seem interested, vote with your feet and find a new dentist.

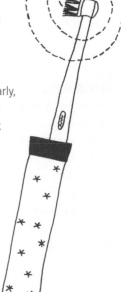

370 BE REGULAR

Brush your teeth regularly, aiming to brush for two minutes, and work methodically around the mouth covering every surface of every tooth. It's better to brush really well once a day than several cursory attempts.

371 BRUSH YOUR TONGUE

Your tongue can be home to many of
the microbes you're trying to get rid of
by brushing your teeth. Your teeth will be
cleaner and your breath fresher if you brush
it with a toothbrush or use a tongue scraper.

372 GO ELECTRIC

One of the best brushing methods for
super-clean teeth is to go electric –
with your toothbrush, that is. Electric
toothbrushes are a great choice because
they don't tire like arms do and are fine-
tuned to stop you brushing too hard.

373 FLOSS WELL

When you floss, don't force the floss
between your teeth. If you have
overcrowded teeth that you can't get
floss into, use flossing sticks instead.
As you floss each gap between your
teeth, slowly move your fingers
along the piece of floss so that
each gap is cleaned by a fresh bit
of floss. That way, you'll avoid
spreading bacteria.

374 GET FLOSSY

Floss once a day between your teeth to
make sure you remove all food debris. Ask
your dentist or hygienist to help you with
technique and try to floss before bed, so
that your teeth are clean for longer.

375 BUY A FLOSS HOLDER

If your fingers are tired, injured or arthritic
and you find it hard to floss your teeth,
invest in a floss holder so that you can
floss without discomfort.

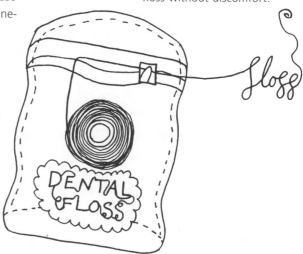

376 PEARLY WHITES

White teeth may be at the top of your list now, but making sure you keep your teeth is more important in the long run. Be sure to see your dentist for deep cleaning.

377 GO SOFT

If your gums show signs of overbrushing, recession or bleed when you brush them, make sure your toothbrush isn't too hard. Choose a soft version, and spend longer gently brushing rather than scrubbing quickly.

378 GET THE BRUSH OFF

Make sure you replace your toothbrush every three or four months, especially if you're using a soft-bristled brush which could be frayed and splayed in that time.

379 THE LONG STORY

If your teeth suddenly start to look longer than they did before, it's possible you're suffering gum recession, which can be a precursor to gum disease. See a dentist immediately, just as you would if you had bleeding gums or a toothache.

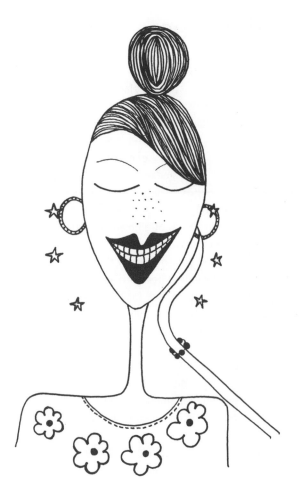

diabetes

380 LOOK AFTER GUMS

High blood glucose helps plaque to grow and people with diabetes can have tooth and gum problems more often if their blood glucose stays high. Smoking is also a risk factor, so if you are diabetic, control your glucose and don't smoke.

381 LOSE WEIGHT

Something like 90% of all diabetes type II sufferers are overweight, and so losing weight is an important part of the care plan. Start by eating slowly to allow your stomach to learn to 'feel full' – chew your food thoroughly and put your cutlery down between mouthfuls.

382 GO NUTS

Nuts are a really healthy food, many containing natural omega oils, but remember they are packed with calories, so try to limit your nut intake to a small handful (about 100 calories) a day if you're trying to lose weight.

383 CHECK YOUR FEET

An early sign of circulation problems due to diabetes is damage to the feet, so make sure you are vigilant about checking your feet for cuts, blisters, sores, swelling or sore toenails.

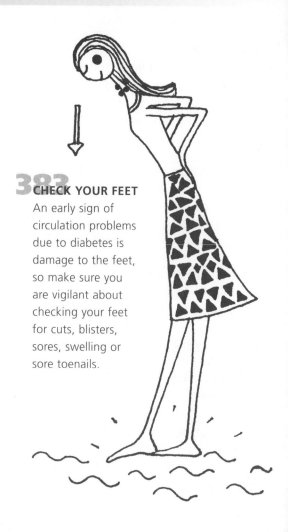

384 GET SWEET AND LOW

If you're diabetic, keeping sugar low in your diet is a must. 'Free' foods contain less than 20 calories and 5 g of carbohydrate per serving, for example, sugar-free jelly, sugarless gum and diet soft drinks.

385 COUNT YOUR CARBS

Sugar-free doesn't mean carb-free or fat-free, so make sure you check labels carefully to see if food is high in carbohydrate even if there is no sugar added.

386 CHECK YOUR LABELS

Remember that fat-free foods can contain almost the same amount of calories as the foods they replace, due to an increase in sugars or carbohydrates. Get label savvy to help your diet stay on track.

387 DRESS WELL

Salad dressing can be packed with calories. Instead of shop bought, make your own with healthy oils like hemp, extra virgin olive or flaxseed, and add mustard and white or red wine vinegar.

388 START EARLY

Research has shown that if you take action to manage your blood glucose before you develop diabetes or when you show signs of pre-diabetes like elevated blood glucose, you can delay or prevent diabetes ever developing through your diet and physical exercise. Take a test to see whether you are at risk and take action.

389 EAT REGULARLY

Diabetics should never miss meals, and the best way to keep blood sugar constant is to eat regularly. Aim for breakfast, morning snack, lunch, afternoon snack, supper and then an evening snack to keep your diet well balanced.

390 CUT THE BOOZE

If you have diabetes, you should try to cut your alcohol intake to as little as possible – replace your usual alcoholic drinks with still or sparkling water or experiment with fruit juices or sugar-free cordials. If you do drink occasionally, never do so on an empty stomach and stick to those low in sugar.

sexual infections

391 DON'T SCRATCH

Vaginal infections can cause intense itching but don't be tempted to scratch as the delicate skin of the vagina can become red and inflamed, which can make matters worse.

392 LOOSEN UP

Avoid prolonged wear of tight-fitting clothes like swimwear, sportswear, tights or skinny jeans, as these can lead to a build-up of bacteria in the vagina.

393 OPEN UP

Although it may be uncomfortable, talk to your partner before having any sexual contact. Ask them if they could be at risk of having an STI and, if necessary, to get checked out. Tell them if you have one too.

394 WIPE AWAY INFECTION

Always wipe from front to back after going to the toilet because improper wiping can spread bacteria to the vagina and is thought to be a leading cause of vaginal discharge.

395 DOCTOR'S ORDERS

When it comes to treating STIs (sexually transmitted infections), it's important to follow your doctor's instructions completely. Not finishing a course of drugs, for example, could mean you are still infected but without symptoms, and you could pass on the infection to your partner.

396 AVOID TOUCHING

You should never touch sores or rashes that you think could be due to an STI. If you do touch one, wash your hands straight away. Always abstain from sexual contact while you are being treated and use a condom when you have sex, even when treatment is finished, until you are sure you're disease-free.

397 CHOOSE COTTON

Always wear 100% cotton underwear if you are worried about smells or discharge – it allows your genital area to breathe, helping the vagina to stay dry. Overnight, give your vagina a chance to breathe by not wearing anything on your bottom half.

398 DON'T DOUCHE

Don't be tempted to douche for the sake of cleanliness as it can actually lead to a higher risk of infections by altering the normal bacterial balance in the vagina.

399 SEEK TREATMENT EARLY

Don't wait to get treated if you think you have an STI – many are easily treated with antibiotics but can cause serious damage if left untreated for too long.

400 LUBRICATE NATURALLY

Don't use petroleum jelly or heavily fragranced oils for vaginal lubrication when you have sex as this can create a breeding ground for bacteria to grow. Try to choose more natural forms such as water-based lubes instead.

401 TAKE A PEE

To help reduce your chance of picking up a sexually transmitted infection, urinate soon after you have sex. Some authorities believe this may help clean away some germs before they have a chance to infect.

premenstrual syndrome

402 DIP INTO DANDELION

To relieve water retention caused by PMS, try putting 10–20 drops of dandelion root tincture in a cup of water with meals and/or before bed. The substance is thought to help the body repel excess water.

403 GET SOME NETTLE

Make yourself an infusion of stinging nettle and drink at least a cup every day when you are feeling the effects of PMS as it is thought to help reduce water retention.

404 ASK YOUR MOTHER

Motherwort is a great herb for calming mood swings, especially for women who feel angry before their period. Try 5–10 drops in a small amount of water several times a day to help you feel calm.

405 TAKE SOME TIME

If you find you suffer badly from the emotional effects of being premenstrual, make a habit of spending some time alone doing something you enjoy at the beginning or end of your period so you will start to create good associations.

406 LIVE IN CLOVER

Taking a cup or more of red clover or mint infusion daily can help to boost your body's level of minerals and vitamins and reduce the tenderness and fluid retention often associated with being premenstrual.

407 CHOOSE CABBAGE

If you suffer from really sore or tender breasts before your period, try the old midwives' remedy of cabbage leaves, steamed whole until just soft, then applied warm directly to the breast.

408 GET YOUR GREENS

Women whose diets are high in calcium and magnesium – found in leafy greens, yogurt, and many herbs – have been found to have less breast tenderness during their menstrual cycle.

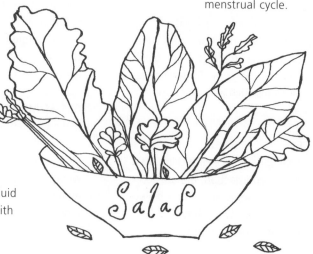

409 GO LIVE

To help relieve constipation and gut problems, which some women get during their period, eat a serving of live yogurt in the morning. This can replace gut flora and help ensure easy digestion all day long.

410 SOW YOUR OATS

For women who feel agitated in the few days before their period, eating porridge or drinking oat milk or an oat straw infusion may help to calm frayed nerves.

arthritis & joint pain

411 DITCH THE COFFEE

Instead of bread, pastries and sugar-filled cereals for breakfast, switch to wholegrain fibre like oatmeal, and fruit or fruit juice and water, instead of coffee and tea. A healthy diet is thought to reduce the effects of arthritis.

412 DON'T IGNORE SYMPTOMS

If you have pain, stiffness or swelling in or around a joint for more than two weeks, you should see your doctor immediately and get a proper diagnosis – early treatment for arthritis can mean less pain and joint damage. Treatment may include exercise, pain management, medication, weight management, dietary advice and instruction on the proper use of joints.

413 RED LIGHT FOR ORANGE

Recent research has shown the importance of vitamin C and other antioxidants in reducing the risk of osteoarthritis. Oranges and other citrus fruits are also good sources of folic acid, which can help alleviate the side effects of the arthritis drug methotrexate, so start eating oranges or drinking juice daily.

414 BE SUN SAFE

Some forms of arthritis, as well as some medications, can make you more vulnerable to the sun, so protect yourself when you go out with sunscreen, clothing and a hat.

415 PROTECT YOUR JOINTS

Losing weight is a great way to reduce stress on joints. You can also protect your joints by using assisting devices and trying to use larger joints for lifting.

416 TRY DIGGING

Gardening has been shown to help ease the pain of arthritis and getting your hands in the soft soil can be really therapeutic. Not only that, but growing beautiful flowers, vegetables or plants will make you feel great.

417 FOLLOW DOCTOR'S ORDERS

Don't mess around with your medication – take it exactly as your doctor prescribes. If you're tempted to stop because it's not working or has side effects, discuss it with your doctor first as it can take weeks or months to settle down.

418 GET MOVING

Exercise helps reduce pain and fatigue, increases range of movement and helps you feel better overall. Your doctor or physiotherapist can show you range-of-motion and strengthening exercises.

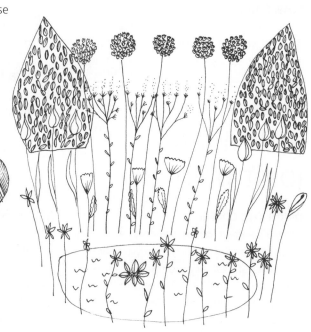

419 REVIEW YOUR MEDICATION

If you've been on your arthritis medication for a while or you feel it's not working as well as it used to, check out some of the new arthritis drugs being developed, or ask your doctor for advice.

420 DRINK MILK

Make sure you include calcium in your diet every day to help prevent bone loss and keep joints healthy. If you don't like drinking milk, try yogurt, cheese and ice cream, or eat leafy greens.

421 GET SHOE-TASTIC

If you suffer from arthritis, wear comfortable padded shoes, which will support your feet and help them to bear your weight evenly, so reducing pain. Walking is the ideal sport for most people with arthritis as it burns calories, strengthens muscles and builds denser bones without jarring joints. Wearing good, supportive shoes or boots is essential.

422 LOOK OUTSIDE YOURSELF

It can be tempting to think about yourself all the time when you're in pain, but looking outside to organizations, charities or causes you believe in and helping others can help reduce suffering by giving you a sense of purpose.

423 EAT WELL

Experts recommend that arthritis sufferers should aim for an anti-inflammatory and low-acidity diet, which means cutting out salty foods such as processed foods, cured meats, bacon, alcohol and sugary foods such as cakes, biscuits (cookies) and sweets (candy).

424 BE HONEST

Don't forget to tell your doctor about any medicines you're taking, including alternative remedies and nutritional supplements, so they can be sure to investigate any possible adverse interactions.

425 SOAK IT AWAY

A warm bath before bed can help relieve muscle tension, ease aching joints and prepare your body for a good night's sleep. Use your favourite essential oil for an added relaxation boost. Lavender, ylang ylang, geranium and chamomile are all relaxing.

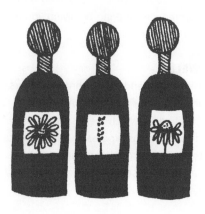

426 SHARE THE FLARE

Don't go it alone if you have a flare up – you'll need to enlist the support of your family and friends if you are going to cope with living with arthritis, and if you're moody they need to know the cause. Learning to communicate effectively with others is key to managing a long-term condition like arthritis.

427 TAKE UP MUSIC

Learning a musical instrument is a great choice for arthritis sufferers – not only does it help keep the fingers flexible (particularly if it's piano or other string instruments) but music has been shown to boost wellbeing and reduce pain.

428 COVER UP

Sometimes, arthritis-related conditions or medication can cause rashes and flushing of the cheeks or tightening or swelling of the skin. Modern cosmetics are great for camouflage, helping not only to cover up but so that you feel better about the way you look and therefore more confident.

429 ICE IT

When joints are hot, red and inflamed, applying a cold pack can decrease pain and swelling by reducing blood flow. A bag of frozen peas is a great choice because it fits well around the contours of the body.

430 GIVE UP THE WEED

Smoking can increase your risk of complications from lupus and rheumatoid arthritis and can predispose your bones and joints to osteoporosis, as well as lengthening recovery from treatment or surgery.

431 HEAD FOR THE HYDRO

Hydrotherapy centres and classes can offer fantastic pain relief and a chance to exercise without restriction. Because the water is warmer than in swimming pools, it can help joints loosen and move. Or sprinkle Epsom salts in your next bath if you want to soothe arthritic pain. It may sound like an old wives' tale but it works!

432 GET GLUCOSAMINE

Studies have shown that glucosamine can improve the symptoms of arthritis if taken in conjunction with chondroitin. Together, the substances are thought to help rebuild cartilage in damaged joints.

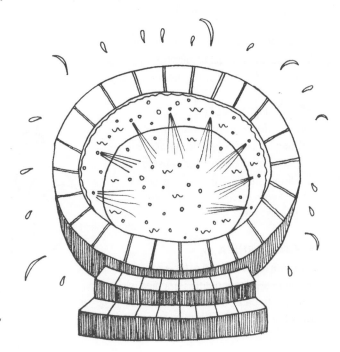

433 BE A FISH

Swimming is great exercise for arthritis sufferers because it is weight-free, meaning joints are supported in the water and muscles can really get to work. And fish oils are a great choice if you suffer from arthritis, as the omega oils they contain are thought to help lessen inflammation and reduce pain. Aim for 225 g (8 oz) of oily fish or 1600 mg of omega-3 supplement a day.

434 GET ALLERGY TESTED

If you suffer from rheumatoid arthritis it's worth getting an allergy test. Common culprits for causing the condition are milk and dairy products, wheat, corn, peanuts, beef, citrus fruits and coffee.

435 ASK FOR ARNICA

If your arthritis started after a fall, one of the best homeopathic remedies is thought to be arnica. Rubbed directly onto the skin, this can also help other types of arthritis as well.

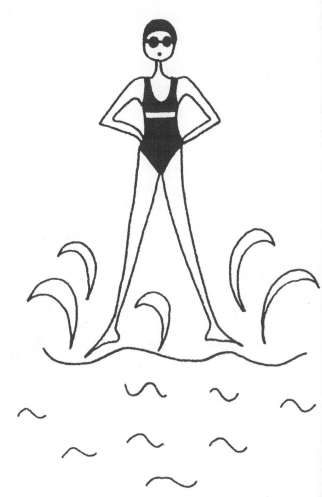

436 GET SOME RE-TOX

To help reduce stiffness in joints caused by arthritis, try the homeopathic remedy rhus tox. But remember to always discuss medications with your doctor in case of contraindications.

437 CLAW BACK

Devil's claw is a herbal remedy which is thought to have anti-inflammatory properties. It is an excellent choice for rheumatoid arthritis, the form caused by inflammation and which is common in men.

438 A RUB DOWN

Getting a massage from a certified professional – or even from a partner or friend if you can't afford a pro – can help reduce pain and inflammation and make you feel good too.

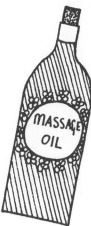

439 BARK AWAY PAIN

If you want a natural herbal remedy instead of taking aspirin for pain, choose white willow bark which comes from the same natural source. Remember to seek advice if you're already on medication.

440 BE A HONEY

To help relieve the symptoms of arthritis, take one teaspoon of cider vinegar and one teaspoon of honey in warm water every morning. The combination is thought to have a soothing effect on sore joints.

441 COOK UP SOME CABBAGE

If you have sore and painful areas on your body from arthritis, try making a homemade poultice from cabbage water or cabbage leaves, which are thought to draw out inflammation and reduce pain.

442 DANCE INDIAN

Indian dancing is a great way to combine exercise with flexibility and strengthening – and, importantly, it targets the hands, which can be useful for arthritis sufferers.

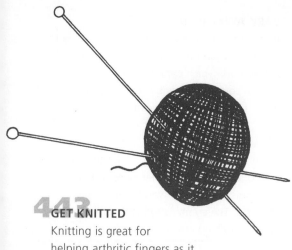

445 BE MAGNETIC

Some people swear by magnetic bracelets or pads to alleviate the pain of arthritis, while others wear them simply to keep it at bay. Remember that it's easier to tell if a natural therapy is helping if you are not taking any pain medication that might interfere with the results.

back pain basics

443 GET KNITTED

Knitting is great for helping arthritic fingers as it encourages them to stay strong and flexible. It is also thought to be relaxing because of the repetitive movements, which can also help to reduce pain.

444 MINERAL MAGIC

Mineral sulphur, often sold in stores as MSM, can provide some relief from pain and stiffness as it is thought that arthritis sufferers may have a deficiency of sulphur. MSM is often mixed with glucosamine.

446 PAIN RELIEF

If you suffer from a bad back, there is some evidence that taking pain relief straight away for the first few days can help reduce long-term pain too, as the body fails to 'learn' the pain pathways.

447 ICE AWAY BACK PAIN

For painful backs, apply an ice pack to the sore area – a medical ice pack is best, but frozen vegetables wrapped in a tea towel will do just as well. If you can stand it, wet the cloth for a colder effect.

448 WARM IT UP

Ice is often a good way to reduce back pain, but if it doesn't work you could try the opposite – a hot water bottle, bath or shower could work, or try alternating ice and heat for best relief.

449 DON'T STOP

Doctors used to recommend bed rest for bad backs, but research shows that this is actually unhelpful. The best thing to do is try to keep moving, even if it hurts a little, to help the spine stay flexible.

450 WALK AWAY

Walking gently is a great exercise for bad backs as it exercises muscles and joints without exerting too much pressure. If it's too painful to walk on land, try walking in water, which can be more comfortable.

451 MOVE AFTER 30

If you've had a bad back recently, keep in mind the golden rule of not staying in one position for more than 30 minutes while your back regains its strength.

452 STRIP THE BED

If you suffer from a stiff back in the morning, take a good look at your bed – if the mattress sags it could be the cause of your problems and it should be replaced.

453 KEEP IT STRAIGHT

The best way to sit down is without bending your back. Bend your knees to help you sit on the chair and use your arms to help you settle into position. Avoid any twisting or bending.

454 AVOID THE BENDS

Instead of bending over the bath or low shelves when you're cleaning, squat or kneel so that you aren't putting undue strain on your back, particularly the lower back. Take regular 'upright' breaks as well.

455 BE UPRIGHT

Use an upright vacuum cleaner and make sure you keep it close to your body so you're not reaching out too far or bending over it, which could put strain on your back and cause injury.

456 ASK AN EXPERT

When it comes to bad backs and neck pain, everyone thinks they're an expert but it will probably pay off in the long run to seek professional help as there are a wide range of possible causes, most of which are treatable.

457 BABY CARE

Bend your knees to pick up a baby – don't twist as it may hurt your back. Similarly, kneel or squat down to talk to toddlers rather than bending down or picking them up.

458 ADJUST THE COT (CRIB)

If you're putting a baby in and out of a cot (crib), adjust the height so you don't have to bend over too far, or choose a bed with a drop-down side so that you don't have to reach in over the bars.

459 BILLOW YOUR PILLOW

To help protect your back while you sleep, don't just use one pillow under your head – use another under your knees, if you are on your back, or between your legs, if you're on your side.

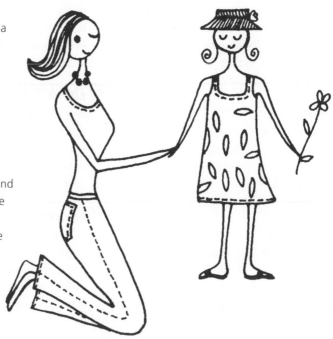

460 KEEP YOUR HEAD STRAIGHT

Lots of pillows might sound luxurious, but really your head should be as flat as possible when you're sleeping, which usually means just one firm pillow is enough.

461 TRY BEFORE YOU BUY

When you're buying a bed, don't fall for marketing ploys like use of the word 'orthopaedic'. Make sure you test out anything before you buy it and choose one that is comfortable for movement as well as lying still. To test if a bed is giving you the right support, lie on your back and slide your hand between your lower back and the mattress. You should be able to work your hand through with a little resistance – too much resistance means the bed is too soft and too little means it's too hard.

462 PUSH NOT PULL

To protect your back from strain when moving heavy items, always push rather than pull an object. Consider the limitations and uses of your anatomy – it help you prioritize your physical wellbeing.

463 STRENGTHEN YOUR ABS

Keeping your abdominal muscles strong will help you avoid back pain. Include stretching in your fitness programme to avoid stiffness, which can cause pain. Pilates, too, is a great exercise to heal, strengthen and stretch the abs and the muscles that support the spine.

464 DON'T TWIST

If you're in pain lying in bed, the easiest way to turn is to bend your knees up and let them fall to one side, allowing their weight to bring your hip and shoulder over. Don't twist.

465 DITCH THE BASKET

When you're shopping, don't lug a basket around the store on one arm, which could strain your back. Put it in a small shopping trolley (cart) until you get to the check-out.

466 DISTRIBUTE WEIGHT

If you're carrying shopping, the best way to protect your back is to use bags with wide handles that you can hold onto easily and then distribute your load evenly on both sides of the body, or use a backpack.

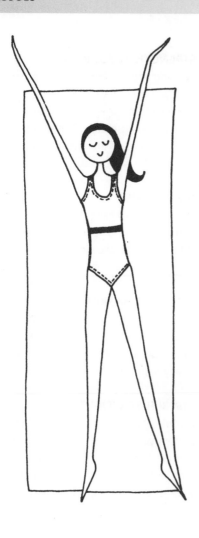

467 STRETCH IT OUT

For at least one minute every hour, take time out from your work to do some quick stretching exercises, even if it's just dropping your head to each side and standing up and stretching out.

468 GET TENS

Transcutaneous electrical nerve stimulation machines (TENS for short) are available from most pharmacies and have been shown to help reduce back pain if used as directed.

469 CHOOSE SUPPORT CAREFULLY

Experts generally believe that using a back support for long periods should be avoided because it can actually reduce back strength. Seek medical advice before using one.

470 A CHAIR STRETCH

To help relieve stress in your office chair, try a quick side stretch by dropping your left ear to your left shoulder while sitting upright, then curling your body over to the left as well. Hold for 30 seconds, breathing normally, and repeat on the right.

471 SIT RIGHT

When using a keyboard, you should aim to sit up with a straight back so that your forearms are horizontal and your feet are flat on the ground. Even if you're comfortable, try to move around every 20–30 minutes.

472 SQUAT IT OUT

Use your office chair to help you stretch out your back between bouts of work. Get out of your chair and hold onto the back of it, then slowly drop down into a squat position with your back straight. Hold and slowly stand up again. Repeat several times periodically.

473 DRIVE AWAY

To protect your back while you drive, make sure your seat has lumbar support, or use a slim cushion. Aim to have your arms slightly bent at the elbow when they are on the wheel. Take regular breaks where you get out of the car and walk around as this will also help concentration and refresh you.

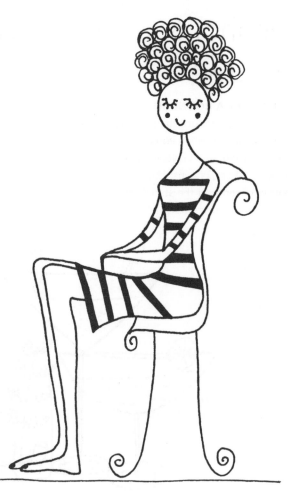

alcohol & drug use

474 DON'T GET A ROUND IN

If you want to reduce the pressure on you to drink alcohol when you're out with friends, avoid being involved in buying 'rounds' of drinks – just buy your own, but tell your friends at the start of the evening so as not to cause offence.

475 AVOID A QUICKIE

Say no to 'quick' drinks, like one at lunch-time or after work. It might not seem like a lot at the time, but over a week it can really cut your overall alcohol consumption.

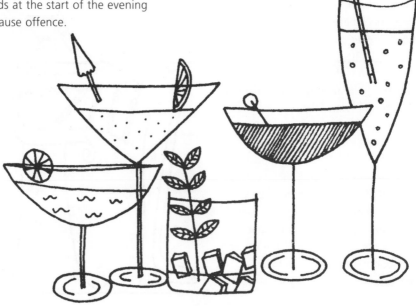

476 GO LOW

If you're worried about drinking too much, replace some of your drinks with low or non-alcoholic drinks instead, or switch your usual drink to one that contains less alcohol.

477 ALCOHOL-FREE DAYS

Aim for at least two alcohol-free days each week. If you find it difficult to do your normal socializing without drinking try something spending your time in a different way, such as developing a new interest or activity.

478 CUT THE SPIRIT

Instead of drinking spirits (liquor), choose longer drinks like beer and wine which contain the same amount of alcohol but take longer to drink.

479 SET YOUR LIMIT

If you have found it hard not to binge drink in the past, make yourself a rule not to have more than a certain number of units, say five – on any single occasion, and don't allow exceptions.

480 MEASURE IT OUT

Home-measuring of spirits and large wine glasses can be pitfalls when it comes to alcohol consumption. Buy smaller glasses, or only fill them halfway, and use a spirit measure to check you're not over-filling.

481 MAKE IT VIRGIN

Instead of only offering people alcoholic drinks when they come to your house, and thus being tempted to have one yourself, why not keep a range of 'special' non-alcoholic drinks, like cordials, iced tea, juice and fizzy water, on hand as alternatives?

482 ASK FOR HELP

Don't try to cut down your alcohol intake in secret – tell your friends you're planning on cutting down so they can support you.

483 TRY SOMETHING DIFFERENT

If you find you're using alcohol as a means of relaxation, actively look for other ways to trigger your body's relaxation response – showers, reading, cooking, relaxation techniques – and sex – can all work.

484 EAT UP

Instead of meeting friends straight from work, go home first and have a meal. Not only will it encourage you to drink less because your stomach will be full, it will also mean you start drinking later.

485 DON'T RUN ON EMPTY

Drinking on an empty stomach is bad news for your liver as well as the morning after. Try to eat before or with your drinks, and if you can't, drink a large glass of milk instead.

486 SEEK ADVICE

If you are worried about your drinking and/or are finding it hard to cut down or stop there are many places to turn for confidential help. Ask sooner rather than later.

487 KEEP A DIARY OF YOUR DRINKING

It can be difficult to keep track of the units of alcohol you are consuming. To get a good idea whether you are within recommended guidelines, write down when, where and how much you drink for two weeks.

488 FIND A SAFE PLACE

Never take drugs or drink to excess in a strange place or somewhere you don't feel is safe as this could be extremely dangerous from a personal safety point of view on top of the risks associated with drug-taking or alcohol use. Make sure you know where you are all the time. Never be alone – be with people you can rely on and make sure you tell them what you've taken so they can help if you get into difficulties.

489 DON'T MIX DRUGS

People combine drugs for two reasons: to make the overall effect more intense or to counteract the unwanted effects of one drug with another – using alcohol or tranquilizers to 'moderate' the effects of cocaine, for instance. But mixing drugs (including alcohol) increases the health risks and means you are less in control. Bear in mind that a combination of stimulants can lead to anxiety, paranoia and increased dehydration as well as putting an added strain on the heart.

490 BEWARE THE COMBINATION

Always avoid taking depressants such as alcohol and tranquillizers together. One of the most dangerous effects of depressant drugs is that they slow down your heart rate and breathing, so if you take them in combination, the risk of overdose and death is significantly increased.

491 AVOID STIMULANTS

Research has shown that taking alcohol and then stimulant drugs like ecstasy or amphetamines increases the risk of heart attack. It's much healthier to drink water, try to sleep off the effects and eat a decent meal when you feel able.

492 DRINK WATER

Whether you are taking drugs or drinking when out in the evening, choose a well-ventilated club and make sure you have access to water to reduce dehydration. Drink at least half a litre (about a pint) of water per hour at a steady rate and make sure you take rests and cool off regularly.

493 FEELING BAD CAN GET WORSE

If you are already feeling anxious, depressed or even just a little bit under the weather, drug or alcohol use can compound your feelings. In the short term you may actually feel physically and mentally worse and in the long term you're more likely to become dependent.

494 STAY PROTECTED

Alcohol and other drugs can make you more relaxed not only about who you have sex with but how you have it. Always use condoms to reduce the risks of unwanted pregnancy and of contracting sexually transmitted diseases, including hepatitis and HIV.

495 DON'T DRUG AND DRIVE

Not only should you steer clear of alcohol if you're driving, you should be cautious about other drugs, including over-the-counter medications. Anything that affects coordination and concentration could be highly dangerous.

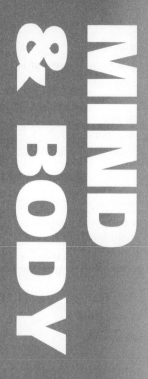

depression

496 DON'T PUT YOURSELF DOWN

Although it's important to be able to recognize your weak areas, instead of just thinking about your weaknesses, match them with strengths to help keep confidence levels high. For instance, if you're impatient, chances are you are also good at adapting quickly to change.

497 WATCH YOUR WEIGHT

A change of more than 5% in your bodyweight in a month, especially if accompanied by sleep changes or feelings of exhaustion, could be a sign you're suffering from depression. Seek help if you're worried.

498 DON'T RUSH IT

If you're being treated for depression, remember it takes time for antidepressants to work. So although you may start to feel better within a couple of weeks, the full effect may not be seen for several weeks or months. Be patient.

499 GET A MASSAGE

It might sound obvious, but it's amazing how many people never get a massage. A treatment doesn't need to cost a lot and having someone take care of you for an hour can make you feel happier and more whole.

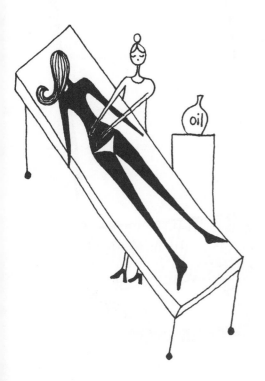

500 CHOOSE YOUR COUNSEL

When you first call a health professional, spend a few minutes asking them questions about their philosophy and approach. Interview several and choose the one you feel most comfortable with.

501 FIND THE RIGHT ONE

If you're having therapy, don't stay with the therapist if you feel the treatment isn't working for you. Review progress regularly and don't be afraid to point out areas you feel could be improved.

502 STRETCH AWAY TOXINS

During the winter, don't neglect exercise. Walking, yoga and pilates are all great ways to keep body's circulation going and alleviate the winter blues.

503 TAKE A CLASS

If you find it difficult to meditate, breathe deeply or concentrate on one thing at a time, consider taking classes in meditation, which could help give you a valuable life tool for relaxation.

504 TRIP THE LIGHT FANTASTIC

Winter is the most important time to make
sure you get some natural light. A walk at
lunchtime is a great way of boosting your
sunlight levels. However, if you suffer from
seasonal affective disorder (SAD), you may
need to buy or hire a light box for regular
exposure to light during dark months. You
need 30 minutes a day at a light level that
you'd get on a clear spring morning, which
is five times brighter than a well-lit office.

505 FIND A PROJECT

Take up a project or hobby that is something
you used to enjoy before you started feeling
down – such as art, politics or volunteer work.
Dedicating yourself to a goal means you don't
have time to think about being sad.

506 KEEP TAKING THE PILLS

Don't be tempted to take yourself off
antidepressants if you start feeling better
without talking to your doctor first.
Continued use under medical supervision
has been shown to lower chances of future
bouts of depression.

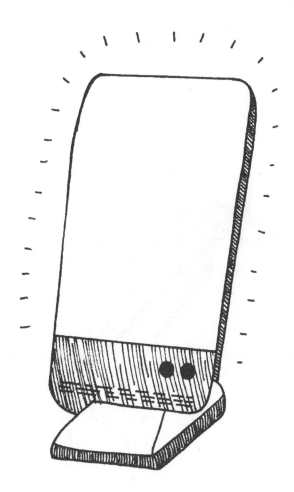

507 KNOW YOUR SYMPTOMS

Depression isn't just about crying a lot or feeling sad. Other symptoms are loss of interest in doing things, changes in appetite and trouble concentrating, sleeping or eating. Seek help if you feel you might be depressed or are suffering from chronic anxiety.

relaxation

508 HAVE A TEA PARTY

Simply going through the motions of making a cup of tea can reduce stress, and each of the four main types of tea (oolong, black, green and white) have their own specific health-giving benefit.

509 TAKE IT WITH YOU

If you're on the move all the time, take a home sanctuary with you. Use a portable basket or case to carry around your candles, oils, reading materials and music so you can create your relaxation area wherever you go.

510 BREW UP SOME RELAXATION

Chamomile, sage, lemon balm and mint can all be used as relaxing infusions. Add two teaspoons of dried herbs to a cup of boiling water and let it brew for a few minutes.

511 GET SOME SPACE

Try to ensure that everyone in the family has their own space, which they can make their own. A bedroom is ideal, but it could also be a corner of a room, a chair or even a shelf if space is tight.

512 RETREAT TO THE SPARE ROOM

If you have a spare room, why not turn it into a sanctuary where you can retreat for a few hours to get away from it all. All you need is a CD player, some candles or incense and maybe even a DVD player, so you can chill out alone.

513 BIG AIR

If you're using candles to help you relax, make sure the room is well ventilated with fresh air circulating so the air doesn't get stale or deprived of oxygen.

514 GET SIDELIGHTS

Light your home to create a sense of comfort and intimacy and think about using different bulbs to provide different moods. Red can help warm up a cold-looking space, and blue can be extra soothing at bedtime.

515 MAKE IT MOODY

Put on a favourite piece of music. It can be something that reminds you of a pleasant memory like a happy holiday or your first romance. Then sit back in a comfortable chair, dim the lights and just listen. The memories you associate with the music will help you relax. Music is also said to appeal to directly to the primal part of the brain to calm and soothe.

516 BE A GUEST IN YOUR OWN HOME

For one night a week, treat yourself like a guest in your own home and lift your spirits with small touches – buy yourself some flowers, change the sheets so they're fresh and use luxurious towels, blankets and toiletries.

517 DO IT ROOM BY ROOM

If you live alone or with a person who shares your interest in relaxation, turn a small area of every room into a relaxation space with a shelf of art objects, floating flowers or some candles. Then you will be reminded of calm wherever you go.

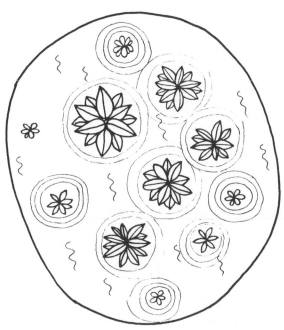

518 THE CHIMES OF FREEDOM

Gentle sounds, such as chimes, can aid
relaxation and act as a reminder to make
your life more peaceful. According to feng
shui, wind chimes can counteract the
negative affects of unnatural sounds, such
as noise from cars and building works.

519 BE BEAUTIFUL

Fill your home with those things that give
you pleasure. Don't worry about conforming
to others' perception of beauty; simply
choose things that appeal to you.

520 SING ALOUD

Singing not only helps you relax because
it feels good, it also helps to regulate your
breathing, which itself reduces stress. So next
time you take a shower, let rip.

521 NURTURE YOUR FRIENDSHIPS

Every couple of months have a night out
with one or two of your closest friends.
It doesn't have to be expensive – just having
a take-away meal at home is a great way to
spend some quality time.

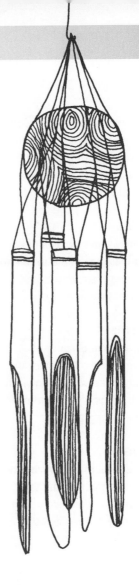

522 OPEN A BOOK

Reading is a great way to escape the stresses of your day, because having the mind focused visually on the words makes it difficult to think of other things. Once a week, turn off the TV and make it a reading night.

523 MAKE THAT CALL

Make one evening a week your phone-a-friend night and really take time to talk to your friends. Sharing your worries and triumphs with friends is important.

524 BATHE AWAY STRESS

Treat yourself to a whole evening of pampering at home. Use a face pack or hair mask in your bath, wrap yourself in warm towels afterwards, do your hair and nails and you'll emerge feeling great.

525 EAT LIKE A KING

Treat yourself to a meal of your favourite food and make it special – set the table with your best cutlery and crockery, dim the lights and really enjoy it. Even if you're on your own you'll feel pampered.

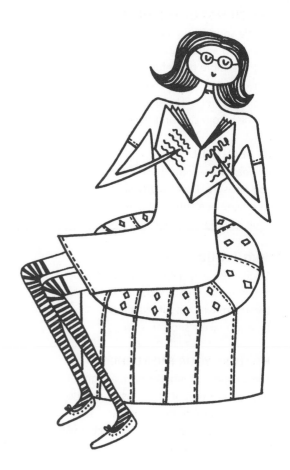

526 AN ORANGE A DAY KEEPS STRESS AWAY

Research shows that vitamin C helps combat anxiety and lower stress hormones. Just one orange provides the RDA of 60 mg and makes a refreshing mid-morning snack. Choose whole oranges rather than juice as they are higher in fibre.

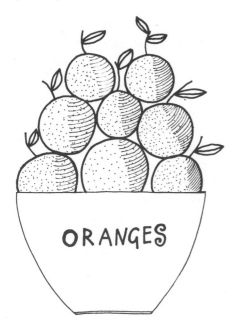

ORANGES

de-stressing

527 LOOK AROUND YOU

For a quick-fix relaxation exercise, if you're out and about, look straight ahead at a wall opposite and just above eye level. Keeping your eyes on that point, begin to broaden your vision so you notice more and more of what's around it. Gradually bringing your attention to the present like this will help your body relax.

528 STRIP OFF

Did you know that nakedness has been shown to help combat stress? Close the curtains, turn up the heating and have some naked time at home to help you feel really free.

529 BAG AWAY ANXIETY

Get a small brown paper bag, squash the top together as if you were going to pop it and breathe in and out through it as slowly as you can for 30 seconds to a minute. Stop if you feel light-headed. It's a great remedy for anxiety, panic attacks and general stress.

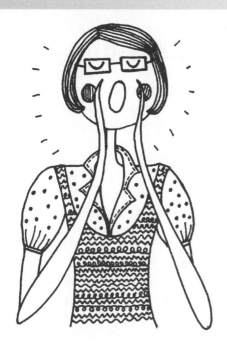

531 DIVE INTO CALM

Many people believe water has spiritual qualities for healing, so a gentle swim is a good choice after an argument or to wind down after a stressful day at work. Swimming is also a particularly good form of exercise because you're weightless in the water, which has positive physical and emotional effects.

532 BUBBLICIOUS ENERGY

Imagine you have a bubble of energy projecting from your central point and surrounding you, like a force field. Give it a colour if you want, and use it to shield you from stress and tension. This is especially good on public transport.

530 WHAT A SCREAM

If you feel the stress building up inside you and don't know what to do about it, take yourself off to a quiet corner and scream it out. Primal screaming has been shown to lower blood pressure and unleash stress and deep-held feelings, so make it as loud and heartfelt as you like.

533 FLOAT ABOVE

In emotional situations, it can be useful to be able to step outside yourself, so let your imagination do just that. Imagine you are floating above your body, higher and higher, until you reach a comfortable point. Then use your new perspective to help you deal with the situation better.

534 AN INVISIBLE FRIEND

Imagine you had an invisible friend who told you all the things you tell yourself during the course of the day. Would you take that kind of abuse? Make your own voice your best friend by striving to be positive. Practise the empty chair technique, where you sit with an empty chair or cushion opposite you, imagine yourself facing you and speak positively to yourself about concerns.

535 DESK MATE

If you often get irate or stressed at your desk, give your hands something to do to help relieve the irritation. Keep a ball or other 'fiddling' toy to hand and use it when you feel stressed, remembering to breathe slowly and relax.

536 GET TO YOUR CORE

To reduce anxiety, concentrate your attention on a point a few inches below your navel and halfway between your front and back. Let your body relax and make sure your knees and jaw are soft.

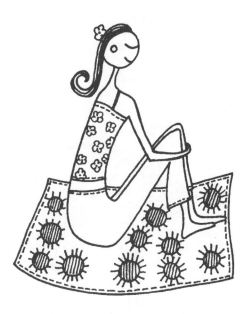

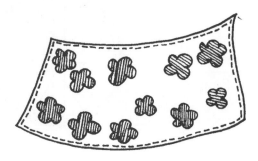

boosting energy

537 PEDAL PUSHERS

Cycling to work is not only good for the environment, it will help you start the day feeling fresh and revived. Exercising in the morning is a great way to boost your system – just don't forget to fuel up with a power breakfast first.

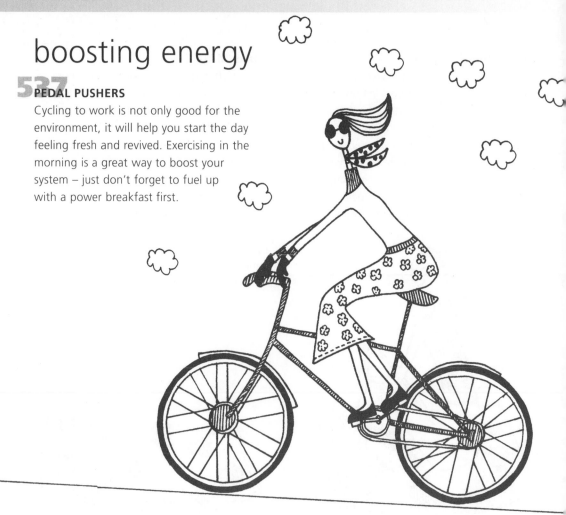

538 DITCH THE CAFFEINE

Give up caffeine – it's a temporary fix and can actually make your brain and body more sluggish and less alert in the long run. Instead, choose water, herbal tea, diluted fruit juice or decaffeinated alternatives to your usual drink.

539 BRAIN FREEZE

If you have a shower in the morning, finish with a two-minute cold burst to boost your circulation and get your scalp tingling. Not only will this wake up your body, it will give your brain a boost of adrenaline to help wake you up naturally, without caffeine.

540 GET WALKING

Walking uses virtually every muscle group in the body and can burn up 520 calories an hour. Not only that, a brisk walk has been shown to flood the body with feel-good endorphins, helping to beat depression and boost mood.

541 BREAK YOUR FAST

Avoid carbohydrates for breakfast and plump for proteins instead to boost your brain's levels of dopamine and increase alertness, as well as keeping your blood sugar steady. Choose eggs, mushrooms, tomatoes or yogurt sprinkled with nuts and seeds.

542 WATER YOUR ENERGY

If you suffer from a late-afternoon slump in energy and concentration levels and have eaten a healthy non-fast-food lunch you are probably dehydrated. Aim to drink around eight glasses of water steadily throughout the day and avoid tea, coffee and fizzy drinks which can add to dehydration.

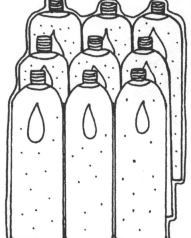

sleeping soundly

543 GET PASSIONATE

If you suffer from sleepless nights, try an extract of passionflower in tea, extract or capsule form. It has been proven to have a mild sedative effect and alleviates nervous symptoms and cramps that can interfere with sleep patterns.

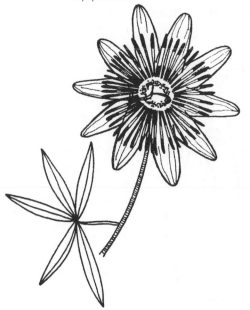

544 FREEDOM FROM CLUTTER

Make sure you always sleep in a room that you find calm and restful if you want to get the most benefit from your night's sleep. For most people that means keeping the bedroom free of clutter, dust, electronic equipment, books, TVs and telephones.

545 WRITE IT DOWN

Keep a pen and paper by your bedside. It can help you in two ways: first, write a list of things you need to tackle the next day; second, write down (and therefore let go) anything that's playing on your mind and that you might find hard to stop thinking about.

546 DO SOMETHING

If you really can't sleep, don't waste time lying there worrying about it. Get up and do something you find relaxing (like reading or watching TV) until you feel sleepy again. You might find going into another room reduces your anxiety about not falling asleep.

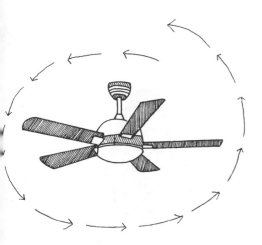

549 SSSSSHHHHHHH!

One of the worst culprits for sleep deprivation is a noisy bedroom. If you live near a road, street or railway make sure your windows are double glazed or well insulated to help reduce noise.

550 DAYLIGHT HELPS

Studies have shown that people who get a good dose of natural daylight every day sleep better at night. Try to get at least 20 minutes outside every day.

547 STAY COOL

Research has shown that people who have fresh air circulating in their bedrooms and who keep the temperature at 18–22°C (65–70°F) have a better night's sleep.

548 KEEP IT MODERATE

Research shows that people who exercise regularly have less sleep troubles, but be careful of exercising late at night. If you must exert yourself close to bedtime, choose moderate exercise like yoga.

551 DITCH THE BOOZE

A small nightcap might help you drift off to sleep more easily, but drinking heavily during the evening is likely to lead to waking in the early hours as your body copes with metabolizing it.

552 GET FRESH FOR SLEEP

Sex is a great way of winding down because it helps relax the body and releases endorphins, which make you feel good and reduce stress.

553 KEEP IT REGULAR

Many people who have trouble
sleeping have erratic time
schedules. Aim to go to bed
and get up at roughly the same
time every day, which will help
train your body's rhythms into
a daily schedule. Taking time to
prepare for bed will also help aid a good
night's sleep by bringing you towards
a state of relaxation.

554 DON'T DRINK COFFEE

Avoid stimulating drinks like coffee,
tea, cola and other drinks containing
caffeine during the evening because they
can prevent deep sleep from occurring.

555 LOWER YOUR SUGAR

Some experts believe that eating foods high
in sugar in the evening can cause waking
during the night as your body's systems
deal with the subsequent sugar crash that
follows. Aim for low-GI foods for your
evening meal.

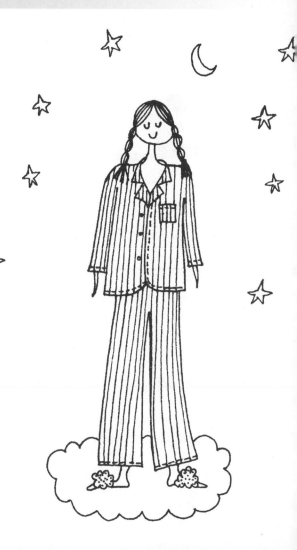

556 B A SLEEPYHEAD

Eating foods that contain lots of vitamin B, such as bananas and avocados, is supposed to help relieve sleep problems caused by adrenal stress. Alternatively, take a B-complex vitamin or the Chinese herb astragalus, which enhances the body's immune function.

557 DIM THE LIGHTS

You naturally come into a light sleep several times during the night. To help you sleep smoothly through them, make your room as dark as possible so the light won't encourage you to wake up.

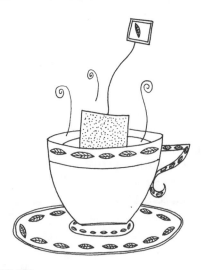

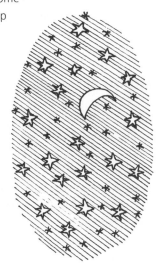

558 HAVE A HERBAL

Although it's best to steer clear of coffee and tea before bed, herbal teas like chamomile and peppermint can relax your system and help you settle down more easily.

559 DITCH THE FAGS

Smoking is bad for sleep because nicotine is a stimulant. Smokers take longer to fall asleep, wake more often and have more sleep disruption than nonsmokers.

560 MAKE IT MILKY

Milky drinks help you sleep because they line your stomach and have a variety of slow-release sugars. Drink them warm for greatest effect but avoid hot chocolate as it contains caffeine.

561 MUSIC ON YOUR PILLOW

Try spending 5 minutes before you go to sleep listening to music as you lie in bed. Helping relax your mind and body in this way will help you drift off to sleep more easily. Nature sounds, such as birdsong, cascading water or wind through the trees, are particularly relaxing.

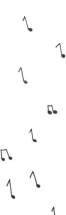

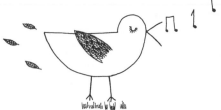

562 BE A LAVENDER GIRL

Sprinkling a few drops of lavender oil on your pillow, or on a handkerchief near your bed, will help you sleep as the herb is linked to restfulness and helps your body feel calm and sleepy.

563 BATH BEFORE BED

A warm bath will gently warm and relax you, and not only that, the corresponding reduction in body temperature about 15 minutes after your bath is a great way to mimic your body's natural sleep rhythms.

564 BEDTIME BREATHING

Spend a few minutes every night before you turn out the lights doing deep breathing while visualizing any areas of tension in your body and releasing them.

565 PLAY A MIND GAME

Counting sheep is the most popular mind game, but anything repetitive will help, like repeating the word 'sleep' over and over again, or imagining walking slowly around a room that is covered in black velvet.

566 BUILD AN IMAGE

Use mental images of a favourite or
fantasy place or moment (such as a
wedding, winning the lottery or an
idyllic holiday spot) as a way of helping
you regain feelings of relaxation and
wellbeing before you drift off.

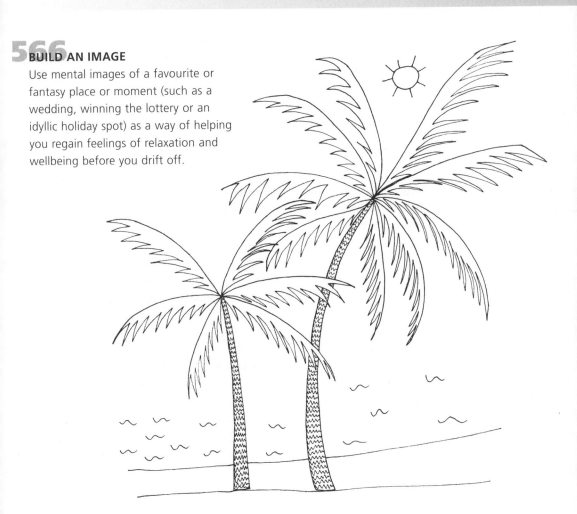

567 CARE WITH PILLS

Be cautious about sleeping pills because although they might help you go to sleep, they do not give you a natural sleep and there is a risk of dependency. If you do use them, it should be for the short term only.

568 TRY TRYPTOPHAN

Foods containing the amino acid tryptophan are thought to help sleep by boosting the brain's natural sleepy chemicals. Turkey, bananas and wholemeal bread are all good tryptophan trips.

take a deep breath

569 BREATHE YOURSELF HAPPY

When you breathe deeply and allow your body to relax, levels of stress hormones reduce in the bloodstream; the more you practise the better your body gets at it. Aim for 10 minutes a day to rejuvenate.

570 FOCUS ON THE BREATH

The best relaxation tip is also the simplest – just close your eyes and focus on your breathing. If your attention wanders, bring it back to your breathing and if you have tension in any part of your body help it relax by breathing into that part.

571 TAKE CONTROL

Changing your breathing is one of the quickest and easiest ways to take control of how you feel. The rapid, shallow breathing we do when we feel fear or anxiety not only makes us more stressed but also lowers immunity and increases susceptibility to heart problems. Concentrate on allowing your breathing to become deeper and calmer.

572 FOLLOW THE SIGHS

For a quick anxiety releaser if you find yourself getting wound up, force yourself to STOP. Breathe in through your nose and then very slowly breathe out. Relax the muscles in your jaw, neck and shoulders as you do so. It only takes a few seconds but can have great benefits.

573 DON'T PANIC

Instead of letting your feelings of anxiety, panic or stress overwhelm you, take control by concentrating on using breathing to help you stay calm. Breathe in and out more slowly and you'll feel you're doing something to help yourself.

anger management

574 LET'S PRETEND

A great way to control your anger if you need help is to pretend you're calm. Projecting an outward vision of calmness will actually help you feel more calm and less angry inside.

575 WALK AWAY

If you are in a situation that is making you angry, leave the room for a while or take a walk. It's easier to think of solutions to problems when you have calmed down.

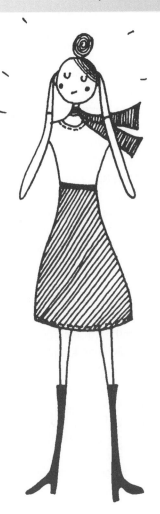

576 EXPRESS YOURSELF

Next time you feel your temper might get the better of you, try to explain your feelings to yourself to get at the root of your anger. Aim to be assertive but not aggressive in your dealings with others.

577 SPOT THOSE TRIGGERS

If you feel your anger is out of control, wait until you're feeling positive and try to think about the things that trigger loss of temper. Then, work out how you could avoid those triggers.

578 PLAY MUSIC TO AVOID ROAD RAGE

Instead of sitting in a silent car with nothing but the sounds of traffic to spark off road rage, listen to your favourite music or the radio to distract your anger.

579 RELAX AWAY RAGE

Gripping the wheel, slouching and arching your back while driving all cause muscles to become tense. Take a moment when you're driving to consciously relax tense muscles and help you remain calm.

580 TAKE A BREATH

When you get angry a big surge of adrenaline goes through your body and your heart rate and blood pressure go up. This causes the reasoning part of your brain to shut off for a short while. Taking a deep breath short circuits this system to help you regain control.

581 SUPPRESS ANGER

If you have anger problems, instead of allowing yourself to fly off the handle the next time you feel angry, make a deliberate effort to quash your feelings. Then, when you have calmed down, you can take that energy and put it to positive use.

582 ALLOW MORE TIME

If you find yourself getting angry when you're driving on particular journeys, allow more time and avoid travelling at high traffic periods. The same applies when you're not driving – always leave plenty of time to allow for delays. One of the most stressful aspects of modern living is being under time pressure.

583 BE REASONABLE

Use words to describe your anger and help you decide if it's appropriate or not. For instance, if someone causes you pain it's reasonable to feel angry, but if they simply get in your way or slow you down it's not.

584 CONFUSED EMOTIONS

Don't confuse anger with jealousy. It's not reasonable to feel angry with someone simply because they have something you don't or are better than you at something.

585 DEFINE YOUR ANGER

Learn to define your problem and face it head-on rather than let it build up. Passively allowing circumstances you are unhappy with to continue will lead to suppressing your anger, which can stop you being able to act to real and serious threats to your wellbeing.

586 ACT, DON'T REACT

Stop reacting to what others say or do, and act positively instead. Changing the situation through deeds, rather than words, is less inflammatory and requires thinking it through.

think positive

587 KEEP A DIARY

Every day for a month, write down ten things for which you are thankful. Choose an attractive bound journal or cover a plain book in photos you love. Not only is it a great way to become a more thankful person, but it's good to read through in your low moments.

588 MAKE ONE GOOD DECISION

Make a decision – today – to change one thing and one thing only. Make the change, then when you've achieved it, think about making another. If you can't face the big changes like stopping smoking, start small by making an extra 10 minutes for your family each day, or limiting your intake of junk food to once a week.

589 BOX UP POSITIVITY

Make a collection of quotes, statements, and compliments about being positive or thankful and keep them in a box. Once in a while, get the box out and read through the quotes to help you feel better.

580 SAY THANK YOU

When people give you
gifts, however small,
send a thank you note.
It can be an email or
text if you're really
pushed for time, but
saying thank you makes you
stop and think about being
grateful, which, in turn,
helps you feel more positive.

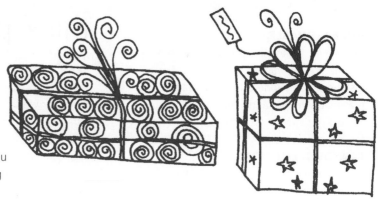

581 ADMIRE YOUR REFLECTION

Make time each week to reflect on the
decisions you have made and how they
have affected your life positively or
negatively. Then make a promise to yourself
to learn from your successes and failures.

582 TIME ALONE

Don't be afraid to let your family and
friends know if you feel you need some
time alone, especially during holidays and
festivities. Be honest and say, 'I could really
do with an hour alone,' then come back
feeling refreshed.

583 LEARN FROM ANOTHER

Find a story about someone who has less
opportunity than you who is nonetheless
achieving satisfaction with life. Use their
story to help you stay positive about your
life and the opportunities you have.

584 GET CLOSE

Close relationships are important for
preventing depression and boosting
wellbeing. Most people have around six
really close friends who can help them in
times of stress, so if you have only one or
two make an effort to enlarge your circle.

595 DON'T LOSE TOUCH

When people are at their busiest and most stressed is often the time they let friendships drop in order to get things done, but it's a false economy. Keep a good balance by making time for your friends, however busy you are.

596 VOLUNTEER

One of the best ways of helping you get a positive outlook on your own life is to volunteer to help those less fortunate than you. Helping out at special needs groups, shelters or hospitals is a good start. Check the local press or the internet for details of voluntary groups.

597 EMBRACE CHALLENGES

It's all too easy to be grateful for things like your house, family and loved ones, but remember to be grateful for life's challenges too. Often, it's facing challenges that helps uncover hidden strengths.

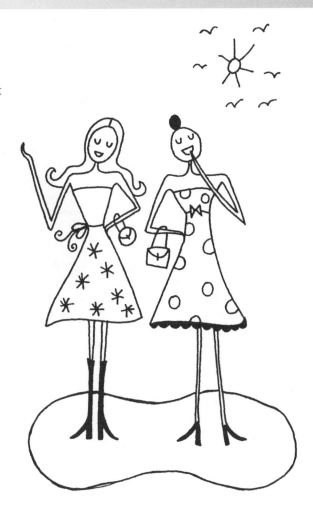

harnessing happiness

598 KNOW YOURSELF

It might sound strange, but spending some time really getting to know yourself could pay huge wellbeing dividends. Identify what it is that makes you really happy and try to make sure every aspect of your life is working towards it.

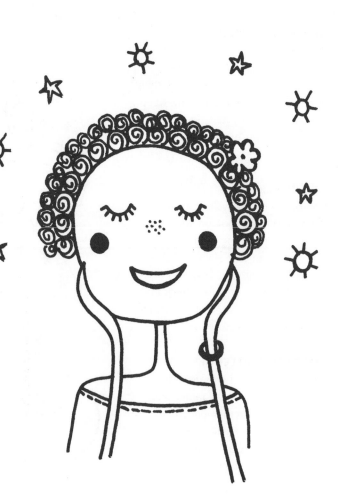

599 TAKE TEN

Try this exercise if you're feeling low or depressed, or if you've got a specific problem you need to solve. Set an alarm for 10 minutes and for that time write or draw continuously about the issue to help you to release hidden insights.

600 USE YOUR WORDS

Next time you feel emotional or overwhelmed by feelings, think about what exactly it is you're feeling. Instead of using words like 'angry' or 'upset', try to think of the reasons behind your feelings, like 'jealous' or 'frustrated'. Knowing your triggers can help you control moods.

601 SAY WELL DONE

Research has shown that people who are enthusiastic and demonstrative with their congratulations when their partner does well at something have stronger and longer relationships, so don't be afraid to let your close ones know when you're proud of what they've done.

602 BE GRATEFUL

Spend some time each day being grateful for what you do have rather than focusing on what you don't have or what has gone wrong. First thing in the morning or last thing at night is often best to help you get your day in perspective.

603 GET ACTIVE

Studies show that people feel less anxious while they are exercising and for the several hours following. It doesn't need to be for long – you only need to exercise for 20 minutes for this natural tranquillizer to kick in. A brisk walk or even some gardening or housework will work.

604 LEARN TO ASK

The times when people feel overwhelmed and really need help are often the hardest moments of life to ask for help. Instead of cutting yourself off and pretending things are fine, allow yourself to ask for, and accept, help and let your friends and family do something useful for you.

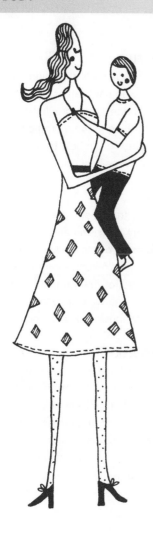

605 LOVE BEFORE MONEY

Research repeatedly shows that loving relationships rather than money lead to people being happier for longer. Don't neglect the people you love in order to make money and be a success. Spend time with your partner, children, parents and friends, making sure they know they are important to you.

606 DITCH THE GREEN MONSTER

Jealousy is a negative emotion and often a hidden one, but it can be very damaging to relationships. Try not to listen to what outsiders say and trust your own instincts. The Bach flower remedy of holly is said to be good for general jealousy and chicory is thought to be helpful if you are jealous of another's possessions.

607 THE PAST IS PAST

Don't let bad experiences in the past put you off trusting friends or partners again – better to risk the occasional let-down than live a life without trusting others, which is seldom happy.

608 LOSE YOURSELF

Think about an activity in which you lose yourself but emerge fulfilled and feeling that you have done well. Try to work out what it is you do right at that time and how you could channel it to other tasks.

609 FIND OTHERS

If you've got a problem you're not sure how to handle and you don't want to share it with friends or family, join a support group. Talking with people who have undergone similar problems can be really helpful.

610 DON'T MISTAKE FINANCIAL SECURITY FOR HAPPINESS

Try to see people's lives and your own as a whole. For instance, your friend might have lots of money, but would you rather swap her single life for your relationship?

611 TRY A REMEDY

If you tend to dwell on emotional hurt from the past that you feel may be holding you back, try the homeopathic remedy natrum mur, which could help you to look forward.

612 FIGHT THE FEAR

If you're a naturally anxious and fearful person, the tendency is to think that everyone else is fearless. To get perspective, ask your friends about what they worry about most and what they are afraid of – remember everyone has something they fear even if they don't show it.

613 START A DISCUSSION

Discuss problems with your partner or friends when things are good between you. It's at these times that misunderstandings are less likely to occur, and you're more likely to sort out problems if neither of you is angry or upset. You are also more likely to see the other's point of view or simply to agree to disagree.

614 STAY TRUE TO YOURSELF

Trying to be – or pretending to be – someone you're not will only lead to anxiety and tension, and people will see through the false exterior. Don't be afraid to be yourself – everyone likes a genuine person more than a wannabe.

embracing change

615 ONE AT A TIME

Don't try to change more than one bad habit at a time, and instead of concentrating on what you haven't done, look at what you have done. Try to replace each negative behaviour with a positive one.

616 THE OCCASIONAL SLIP IS OK

If you're committed to changing a bad habit, don't worry if you slip every now and again – but make sure you don't get lax and allow too much slippage, or allow yourself to let slips be a reason to give up.

617 COME UP WITH A SLOGAN

Using a positive slogan can help you harness the power of habit because repetition of a phrase hardwires it into your brain. Create a slogan such as 'stay on track' or 'one step at a time' and repeat it ten times a day to burn the thought into your brain.

618 ASK ADVICE

Talk with your partner or a close friend about how to reward your good behaviour if you quit a bad habit – keep the reward reasonable and achievable and stick to it.

619 THE RIGHT SUPPORT

Before you discuss making a life change with someone, make sure you are choosing someone who will be supportive. Don't ask a smoker for support on giving up, for instance!

620 GIVE YOURSELF A CHANCE

If it was easy to kick bad habits nobody would have any, so accept you may be in it for the long haul. Chart your progress so that you can see how things develop over time and look back to motivate yourself.

621 MOVE YOUR NOTES

Posting motivational notes around the house to remind yourself to be positive is a great idea, but keep in mind that after a few days your brain will 'background it' unless you move it to a new place.

622 KEEP THE CHANGE

To help you form a positive new habit, put ten coins in your left pocket and each time you remember to do your chosen thing, move one to the right pocket. When you have moved all ten several days in a row, the habit is formed.

623 DO IT FOR THIRTY

Focus on one change only for 30 days and during that time concentrate solely on that one thing and don't try to change anything else about your life. After 30 days, move on to the next change, or take a break from change for a while. Trying to focus on several things is difficult and makes it more likely you'll give up on all of them.

624 PULL THE TRIGGER

Come up with a trigger, which is a short ritual you link with a change to condition new patterns of behaviour. Examples include snapping your fingers every time you want a cigarette if you're trying to quit, or jumping out of bed as soon as the alarm starts if you're used to sleeping in.

625 KICK BUT

Use the word 'but' to help you change negative thought cycles. If you find your inner voice telling you you're bad at something, use 'but' to make it positive like, 'I'm crap at this … but if I keep practising I'll get better'.

626 PRINT YOUR PROMISES

If you've made a commitment to yourself to change, don't keep it in your head where it could become warped or forgotten. Writing down promises makes them harder to break.

627 KEEP SCHTUM

Studies have shown that people who talk about things to exhaustion before they do them are less likely to follow through. By all means discuss your chosen course of action, but don't let words take over from actions.

628 BET ON IT

Motivate yourself to make a habit change by having a wager with a friend. Making a public commitment and promising to give up something you will miss is a great motivator for the low times.

629 BE CONSISTENT

Make sure your habit is as consistent as possible and doesn't require thought or attention. Keeping it consistent will allow the habit to be drilled into your subconscious instead of you having to remind yourself.

630 REPLACE LOST NEEDS

If you're trying to give up a habit that gives you something, like comfort eating or watching television to relax, bear in mind that the feeling you're giving up will need to be replaced with an alternative behaviour.

631 STAGGER YOUR REWARDS

If you're trying to reinforce behaviour, plan to reward yourself as often as possible the first week, then every week for a month and then every month for three months.

632 DO THE CAN CAN

Be vigilant in your hunt for negative thoughts, like 'I can't do it', and keep squashing them and replacing them with positives like 'I can do it; I am doing it'. If you think positive, you will succeed.

633 KEEP IT SIMPLE

Don't let your behaviour change become too complicated. Keep it to a few rules to help form habits and avoid confusion. Exercising every day for half an hour is easier to remember than a complicated weekly regime, for example.

634 MAKE LINKS

Try to link your rewards to your behaviour change. If you're replacing smoking with exercise, for example, use the money you would have spent on cigarettes to buy yourself new exercise gear, a gym membership, or a sports massage.

being a better you

635 SAVOUR THE SMALL STUFF

Allow yourself to enjoy small pleasures each day. Take a walk, sing in the car, have a glass of wine, read your favourite magazine or do whatever it is that relieves stress and leaves a smile on your face.

636 TRAIN THE BRAIN

There are many books, puzzles
and even computer games on
the market that can help keep
your brain active with brain
training. Or simply aim to
learn a new thing every
week to keep your grey
cells working effectively.

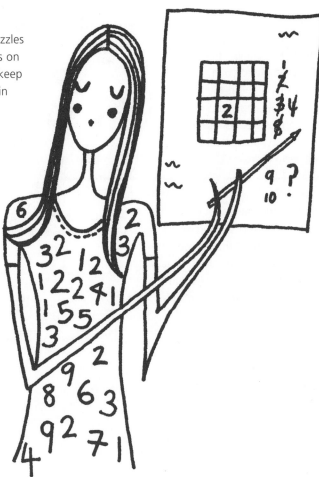

637 BE POSITIVE

For every negative thing you hear yourself say, try to think of three positives. For example, if you hear yourself complaining about the rain, remember how important rain is for modern life as well as nature, and how it makes you appreciate the sunshine even more.

638 MAKE A CHANGE

People who are concerned about their stress levels are less likely to exercise and more likely to be smokers than those who don't smoke and lead active lives. Instead of worrying about your bad habits and the problems they cause, make some positive lifestyle changes.

639 GET A GOAL

Set yourself a goal – be it with relationships, work or home – and make a list of the steps you'll need to take to achieve it. Anything is do-able if you break it down into small enough steps and take each one at a time.

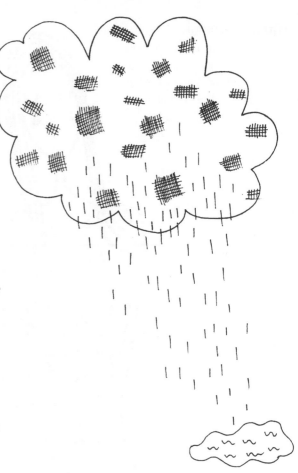

640 MAKE UP YOUR MIND

Unresolved decisions are very stressful. Most decisions are reversible, but getting back time you waste by not making a decision isn't, so be decisive and help reduce stress.

641 FIND A PLACE

Locate a place near to your home which you can use as a relaxing getaway. Whether it's a museum, riverbank, café or the beach, it's good to have somewhere you can take yourself to think things through.

642 TAKE RESPONSIBILITY

Don't plead helplessness when it comes to your life not being perfect. Acknowledge that it's partly down to you and the choices you have made and are making and then do what you can to change them.

643 BE DECISIVE

What's holding you back? Are you waiting for someone to hold your hand, the children to grow up, a lottery win? Being decisive means doing something to enhance your life now, not hanging on for a dream future.

644 AVOID COMFORT EATING

One in four people is thought to turn to food to help alleviate stress or deal with problems, but it rarely works – comfort eaters report higher levels of stress, fatigue and sleeping problems. Try something else instead.

645 DON'T GRAB AND GO

Stress levels are higher among frequent fast-food eaters than those who eat more natural foods. Make time to cook your own meals and eat them at home.

646 KNOW THE DIFFERENCE

Women dealing with stress report nervousness, wanting to cry or lack of energy while men talk about trouble sleeping or feeling irritable or angry. Understand the differences to help support your partner in times of stress.

647 SHARE THE BURDEN

Stress is higher for the family's health-care decision-maker, which in 75% of families is the mother. Try to share decisions with your partner to avoid piling on the stress.

acupuncture & acupressure

648 POP A PLACEBO

The placebo effect is powerful – it often works even when we know it's a placebo. Even if you don't totally buy into alternative remedies, they can still work for you, so don't be afraid to try something you're sceptical of.

649 DON'T BE LATE

Many complimentary therapies, including acupuncture, are most effective if you are calm and unstressed. To help achieve an unstressed state, arrive ten minutes early so you have time to relax before treatment.

650 NOSTRIL RELEASE

To release nasal 'stuffiness', push down directly below the outer border of each nostril, on either side of the base of your nose. Feel for a small indentation (flaring and relaxing your nostrils can accentuate the point) and press into the point equally on each side for five minutes.

651 GET STUCK IN

Research shows that acupuncture can help a range of conditions, including pain, premenstrual tension, stress and insomnia as well as anxiety and depression. It works by balancing flow of *chi* (the 'life force') through the body. But make sure you see a trained and licensed professional.

652 BE UPFRONT

To get the most out of your acupuncture treatment, it's important to start off on the right foot. Tell the acupuncturist about any medical conditions, drugs or problems you have and if you are, or could be, pregnant.

653 MAKE YOUR POINT

Choose your acupuncturist carefully – make sure they belong to your country's professional register and that you feel comfortable with them. Don't be embarrassed about asking questions, especially if you have specific conditions you want treated.

654 TREAT ADDICTIONS

There is increasing evidence to show that visiting an acupuncturist could help to overcome addictions like alcohol and smoking by reducing cravings and instilling a sense of wellbeing.

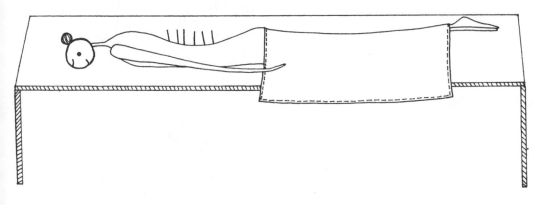

655 GET SOME YANG

One of the telltale signs of stress is also an acupressure trick for reducing it – massage your temples in slow, circular motions with flattened fingers. Breathing deeply and closing your eyes can help accentuate the result.

656 STICK YOUR TONGUE OUT

Drinking and eating before an acupuncture appointment could affect the natural coating of your tongue, which is often used to help diagnosis. Similarly, don't brush your teeth or use a tongue scraper beforehand either.

657 WHEEZE AWAY WITH PRESSURE

To help reduce wheezing for asthmatics, cross your hands over your chest and using your fingers to press down on the middle point between neck and end of shoulder for a few minutes (don't do this if you're pregnant).

658 KEEP IT LOOSE

If you're going to see an acupuncturist, make sure you wear loose clothing that you'll feel comfortable lying down in. This will also help you feel comforted afterwards.

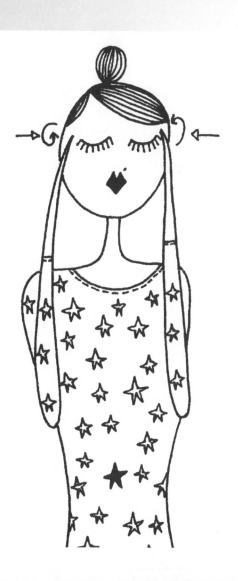

659 DON'T FILL UP

Before you have acupuncture you should avoid large meals, alcohol, coffee and smoking, which may change the 'pulses' your acupuncturist will feel for in order to choose the right treatment.

660 BE QUIET

After you've visited an acupuncturist, it's sensible to build in 20 minutes or so of quiet time to allow yourself to 'come back' to your normal life pace. Many clinics have rooms where you can do this.

661 PRESS IT OUT

If you're performing self-acupressure and your fingers get tired, use the rubber (eraser) end of a pencil or the thick end of a chopstick instead.

662 PINCH YOURSELF

If you start to feel light-headed or tired, pinch yourself on the very centre of the tip of your nose. Hook your index finger over the 'bulb' of your nose to anchor it, then dig your thumbnail in firmly.

663 HEAL YOUR SCARS

Promote healing with moxibustion, the therapy of burning herbs at acupressure points, often used in conjunction with acupuncture. For recent scars (allow eight weeks of initial healing) wave a lit moxa stick (available from Chinese therapists) a few inches above the scar site to warm the area and restore good *chi* flow.

664 MASSAGE AWAY JAW PAIN

To help relieve jaw pain and toothache, use your thumb to massage small circles into your acupressure point in the base of the fleshy valley where your other thumb meets the fingers (do not do this if pregnant).

665 PRESS AWAY INSOMNIA

When you can't get to sleep or you're restless, massage underneath the bony ridge around the back of your head, working your thumbs under the ridge line from the ears to the centre above your neck. You can also apply steady pressure for three minutes, using several fingers, to the point on the inside of the wrist crease, in line with the little finger.

massage & self-massage

666 TOUCH BASE

To relieve a tense neck and shoulders, try this self-massage tip: make small circular movements with your fingertips, on either side of your spine, working up the neck and around the base of the skull to ease away spasms in muscles.

667 A TIGHT SQUEEZE

One of the most effective ways to reduce tension and spasm in muscles is to go for the squeeze. Apply pressure to the muscle – your shoulder, say – and hold for several seconds, then let go. Work around a whole area.

668 CIRCULATION POUND

A great circulation booster if you've been sitting at your desk too long is to use a loosely clenched fist to gently work the muscles of your opposite shoulder. Keep the wrist flexible and avoid applying too much pressure.

669 GET YOUR FOOT IN

Resting one foot on the opposite leg, put one hand on the top of the foot and the other on the sole and gently work your fingers into the muscles to relieve tension. Better still, get your partner to do it for you.

670 A LEG UP

Knowing how to massage your own legs is really useful for athletes to help post-exercise recovery. It also boosts lymphatic drainage and is thought to help reduce cellulite. Work from ankle to thigh.

671 DEAL WITH CRAMPS

If you are prone to night cramps, giving your legs a massage before bed to boost circulation may help. Stroke the whole leg from ankle to thigh three to five times and knead gently into the thigh and calf.

672 STROKE AWAY NECK PAIN

To help a stiff neck, stroke your right shoulder with your left hand, starting at the base of your skull and ending at the elbow. Repeat three times then do the other side.

673 GET AN AROMA DURING MASSAGE

It might sound like a 'lightweight' therapy, but when you consider that it takes around 20 kg (45 lbs) of rose petals to create just a single teaspoon of essential oil, it's worth giving aromatherapy a try, particularly for stress release treatments. Aromatherapy diffusers release the oils into the air, enabling you to breathe them in during a massage.

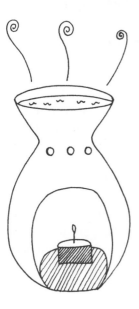

674 STRETCH IT OUT

Most of the things we do with our hands – particularly at keyboards – are contractions, so make sure you take time to stretch them out as well. Spread out your fingers and open the palms as far as possible to stretch them out.

675 FEEL THE PRESSURE

Pressure points in your skull can help relax your whole body. To work them, put two tennis balls in a sock and tie the end. Lie on your back on the floor with the sock behind your upper neck so that each ball touches the part of the skull directly above the hollow spot. Relax for at least 5 minutes, preferably 15 to 20.

676 EAR WE GO

A great tension reliever if you only have a few minutes is to use your ears to help relax your face and jaw muscles. Pull the sides of your ears outwards, then up and down, then use your index finger to press behind the earlobe where it attaches to the head. Hold for several seconds and release.

677 FACE UP TO IT

Don't forget your face when it comes to self-massage. Our faces hold much of the tension of our bodies so make sure you gently work your fingers and palms over it to bring warmth and relaxation.

678 RUB YOUR KIDNEYS

Give yourself a quick energy boost if you're feeling low by rubbing the area above your kidneys – push your fists gently into your back either side of your spine at waist level and rub in a circular motion.

679 NATURAL PAINKILLER

Massage is a great choice for pain relief because it is thought to interfere with the brain's pain signals as well as causing the body to release endorphins, its natural painkillers.

680 THE HEALING TOUCH

Research shows that even a touch from someone else lasting a single second can help people feel better. Ask a friend or partner to help you if you feel you need another's touch.

681 KNUCKLE FOOT PAIN

If your feet are painful at the end of the day and muscles feel fatigued and tense, use a loose fist to make knuckling movements all over the sole of your foot, which helps muscles relax.

meditation

682 SAY THANK YOU

Get into the habit of feeling grateful for the opportunity to do a meditative practice and your mind's ability to focus. Spending a few minutes being grateful at the end of a session will help reinforce the positive effects of meditation.

683 KEEP GOALS IN MIND

The goal of meditation is to create mental space so that your subconscious mind can come to the surface, and to promote a positive outlook and feelings of happiness. Remember this while you practise and the meditation will be more fulfilling.

684 PICTURE HAPPINESS

Your safe place doesn't have to be real; you can create a safe haven for meditation in your mind by picturing a happy place where you feel comfortable and 'going' there when you feel stressed.

685 KEEP PRACTISING

Meditation is a skill and, like any other skill, practise makes perfect. Don't expect to be able to do it straight away, but practise regularly and soon it will be second nature.

686 BE ACTIVE

It's easy for beginners to think meditation is the same as going to sleep, but it is an active process. The art of focusing on a single thing takes hard work and practice, and requires commitment.

687 DON'T ALLOW FRUSTRATION

If you're just starting to learn meditation, frustration is common as thoughts crowd in and threaten to overwhelm the desire for quiet. Focus on the breath if this happens, which helps link body and mind.

688 TAKE IT WITH YOU

If you're just beginning to learn meditation, try it throughout the day by generating small moments of awareness (at your desk, walking through the park, and so on) to strengthen the mind and promote calm.

689 LIGHT A CANDLE

Meditating with your eyes closed can be difficult, as thoughts can crowd in. To strengthen your concentration, try lighting a candle and using it as your point of focus.

690 BRING A FRIEND

Meditating with someone can have many wonderful benefits and can help you both improve your practice. Make sure you set rules before you begin so you both know what to expect.

691 BE AN EARLY BIRD

A great time to meditate is in the early morning when there is a natural quiet and the body is well rested. Ideally you should get up half an hour early, do a few stretches then begin your practice.

692 STRETCH IT OUT

Stretching loosens the muscles and tendons, allowing you to sit more comfortably, so gentle stretching or yoga is a great pre-meditation choice, as is a brisk walk or swim.

693 LEAVE THOUGHT BEHIND

The goal of meditation is to go beyond the mind – it can't be done by thinking alone, we have to help our minds become quiet before they can really relax. Do this by acknowledging thoughts but not allowing them in – picture yourself turning them away from your 'quiet space'.

694 NOTICE YOUR BODY

A great practice for beginners is to take notice of the body when a meditative state starts to take hold. Put all your attention to the feet and then slowly move your way up the body, becoming aware of each part in turn.

laughter

695 CUT THE NEGATIVES

If you've got friends who always leave you feeling low or depressed, try to spend less time with them and more time with someone who makes you laugh and feel good about yourself. If a negative friend always has that effect on you, you may need to reevaluate the friendship.

696 FEED YOUR HUMOUR

Instead of watching heavy dramas that leave you feeling wrung out, spend at least one night a week watching or listening to a comedy programme, sitcom or stand-up.

697 CREATE A FUNNY BOX

Take a box (an old shoe box will do) and use it to store things you find funny, like old cards and cut-outs from magazines, or even DVDs or audio comedy. Dip into it when you feel in need of a boost.

698 HAVE A LAUGH

A recent study by the University of Maryland Medical Center found that people with heart disease were 40% less likely to laugh, and watching a funny movie boosts the flow of blood to the heart in the same way aerobic exercise does. Every day, make a conscious effort to read or watch something funny.

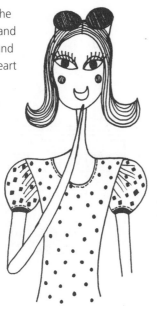

feng shui

699 SOOTHE YOURSELF

Use colours to help create a feng shui sanctuary in your bedroom. Opt for colours which mimic the natural human skin – from pale pinky white to rich chocolate brown.

700 CLOSE YOUR DOORS

Keeping bedroom doors closed at night – including those to en suite bathrooms and walk-in closets – will allow for the most nourishing flow of feng shui energy.

701 BLACK AND BLUE

The feng shui colours of water are black and blue. They are used to help create abundance, including good health. Use them in the north, east and southeast areas of your home.

702 GET FRESH

Open your bedroom windows often or use an air purifier to keep your bedroom fresh and full of oxygen. Plants are good for air quality but try not too have them too near the bed.

703 THE BEDROOM YOU DESIRE

Everyone has different tastes when it comes to décor, but keep in mind two keywords when you are creating your bedroom: pleasure and dreaming. Everything you put in your bedroom should reflect the desire for love, relaxation and healing sleep.

704 CREATE SOME BED SPACE

The best place to have your bed according to feng shui is where it is approachable from both sides, with bedside tables on each side to balance and declutter. Do not position the bed directly in line with the door. A firm mattress, solid headboard and sheets made with natural fibres are all good for creating harmony.

705 GO EAST

To boost health with feng shui, try to incorporate wood or water features in the east of your space (concentrate on your main living area and your bedroom in particular). If you don't want wood or water, choose art that depicts them.

706 THE FIRE IN YOU

A real fire reminds us of our primal energy and warmth but keep the area in front clear so the energy can radiate out. If you can't site a fire or woodburner at the northeast and southwest spaces of your home, as feng shui suggests, try to incorporate some fire colours like red, orange, purple and pink.

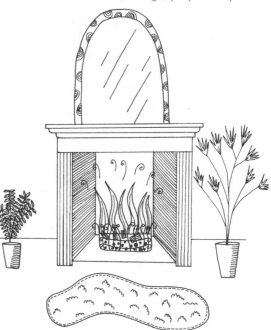

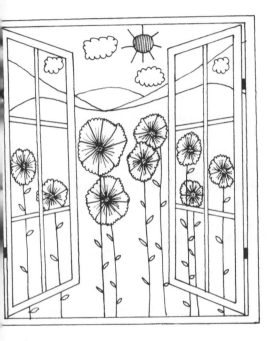

708 BE FRESH

When you're using feng shui techniques to help harmonize your home, the important elements are fresh air, light and a lack of clutter. Concentrate on these three before you embark on specific changes.

709 BE METALLIC

If you want to boost your clarity and precision, try to incorporate some of the feng shui metal elements to the north and west areas of your space. Use metal or grey and white colours.

710 DIM THINGS DOWN

A great way to make your bedroom feel relaxing is to use a dimmer or have lots of different levels of lighting. Candles are great but they're not always appropriate, so other means of low-level lighting are useful.

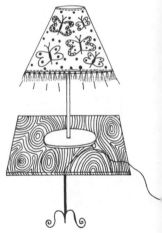

707 ROOM WITH A VIEW

According to feng shui, the most important views to concentrate on are the view from your bed and the first view you see when you walk in the door. Make sure these are attractive and clutter free.

711 GET A GOOD IMAGE

Make sure the paintings and prints you choose for your bedroom reflect what you want to see happening in your life. Avoid colours that clash or anything violent or too bright. Nature scenes such as landscapes are calming and relaxing.

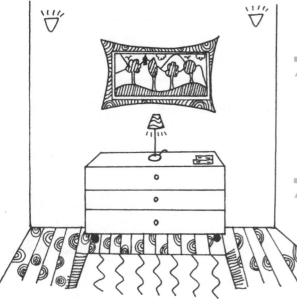

yoga

712 GET TOASTY

If you're meditating at the end of a yoga or pilates session, make sure you keep yourself warm with a blanket or shawl. Being still and reducing heart rate with deep breathing after exertion can cause the body temperature to drop, and that will reduce your ability to relax.

713 MAKE A CHOICE

Read up on different types of yoga before you pick one that is right for you. For most complete beginners, a Hatha or Vinyasa class will be most appropriate as they are least demanding physically.

714 EAT LIGHT

Don't have a big meal before a yoga class as this could affect your energy levels and give you a cramp. Aim to eat light meal a few hours before the class is due to start and drink water to stay hydrated.

715 GO BARE

It's best to take off socks and shoes and to practise yoga in bare feet as many of the postures involve your feet being aligned properly and being aware of the ground. If your feet get cold you can wear socks during relaxation, though.

716 DO LIKE A DOG

The Downward Dog yoga position (with hands flat on the floor, feet flat or heels pressing down towards the floor and bottom in the air to form a triangle) is great for clearing your head of stressful thoughts. It helps reduce blockages in the neck and shoulders and allows blood flow to the brain.

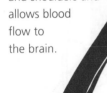

717 GO AT YOUR OWN PACE

Whenever you're doing exercises at home like stretching, pilates or yoga, pay attention to pain. Do things at your own pace and never be tempted to push yourself too far to keep up with someone else.

718 SPEAK OUT

The first time you attend a yoga class make sure you tell the teacher and, if possible, choose a place near to them so that they can keep an eye on you.

719 HOT TO TROT

Bikram yoga is a series of exercises practised in a heated room. As you can imagine, a vigorous yoga session at high temperatures promotes profuse sweating and loosening of muscles. It is said to be cleansing and to rid the body of toxins but it is not for beginners. Make sure you drink plenty of water before and after the class and don't eat for two hours beforehand.

730 DRINK UP BEFORE

Because yoga is designed to have beneficial effects to your internal organs as well as the muscles and bones of your body, it's a good idea not to drink water during class – but make sure you top up before and after.

721 YOGA FOR LIFE

A holistic therapy, yoga heals the mind, body and spirit. Yoga means 'yoke' or 'union' in Sanskrit and its aim is to integrate all the various aspects of your life so that your mind and body work together.

722 GET INTENSE

If you're an active person who enjoys exercise, Ashtanga yoga might be the right choice as it is an intense style based on constant movement, or flow, from one pose to the next. Attend a beginner's class first.

723 HOLD THE POSE

If you are a naturally precise person, you will probably enjoy Iyengar yoga, which is a style based on postural alignment that concentrates on holding poses for a long time.

724 GET INTERACTIVE

If you enjoy being social and want your yoga practice to be spiritual as well as physical, Kundalini yoga is a good choice because it concentrates on the breath and often involves chanting.

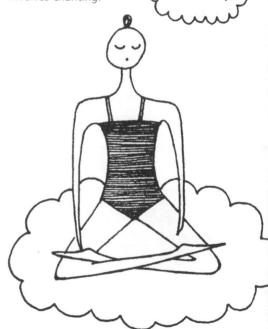

OM!

725 STAY UNSTIMULATED

If you're new to yoga, the effects can be
fairly dramatic. Avoid energizing and
stimulating postures like the Sun
Salutation and standing Warrior poses in
the evening. Try practising slow forward
bends and the prone Corpse pose, which
creates a deep state of relaxation.

726 DON'T PUSH IT

While it's natural – and often helpful –
to look around you in a yoga class to see
what everyone else is doing, don't worry
if they seem to be able to do more than
you. Everyone's bodies are naturally
different and it's dangerous to try and
push yourself. You'll feel the benefit
whatever your level.

727 ALL OR NOTHING

If you are the type to throw yourself
into something wholeheartedly, choose
Sivananda yoga, a form of Hatha, which
is based upon the five principles of
proper exercise, breathing, relaxation,
a vegetarian diet and meditation.

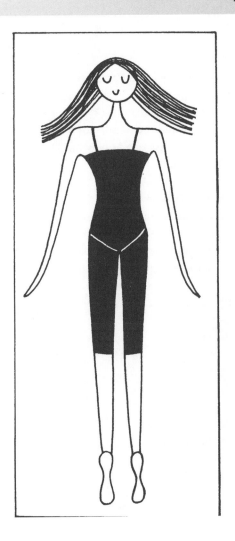

728 KEEP AT IT

You will probably feel a bit stiff or sore after your first yoga class, especially if you don't take regular exercise, but stick at it for a few weeks before you decide not to go back – you'll be amazed at how quickly your body adapts.

729 HAVE A HATHA

If you're a naturally relaxed person who likes taking things slowly, a Hatha yoga class is probably for you as it's likely to have a slow pace and provide a good introduction to basic poses and breathing exercises.

730 HANG LOOSE

If you're practising yoga at home, even if you're a beginner, be sure to wear clothes that allow for freedom of movement but which are not so baggy that they could restrict flow. Lycra and cottons work well.

731 KEEP IT CLEAN

The ideal setting for doing yoga at home should be well ventilated, have natural light and be free from distractions and interruptions. Turn off phones and practise on a carpet or a mat that is long enough for you to stretch out on.

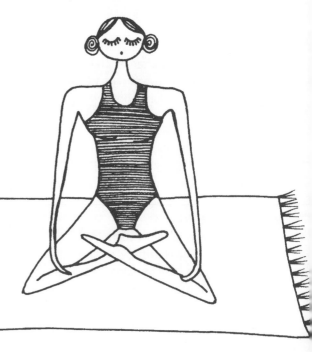

732 STAY BALANCED

If you're trying yoga poses that involve balance, put a 'focus' object a few metres (yards) away from you to fix your gaze on as you balance. A painting or photo at eye level is best, but a plant or even a pile of clothes will do.

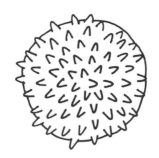

733 RUNNING ON EMPTY

Dedicated yogis will only perform exercises on an empty stomach, but there's no real evidence that this makes it easier or gives greater benefits. As with any form of exercise, it's sensible to avoid doing any moves straight after a large meal, though.

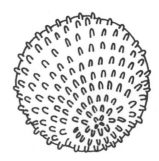

reflexology

734 HOLD YOUR HEELS

For a home reflexology treatment to help problems in the pelvic area, try massaging your heels or rolling them around on a soft ball. The heel of the foot is linked to the pelvic area so it's a great place to target if pregnant.

735 EASE BREATHING

To help ease breathing problems, relieve stress and relax the chest and ribs, stand on or roll your foot over textured reflexology or massage balls (or golf or tennis balls if you don't have any to hand) in the centre of your foot at the toe end of the arch.

736 TOE THE LINE

The bottom of the big toe in reflexology is thought to link to the hormone-controlling pituitary gland, so if you're feeling low and think it might be hormonal, or if you're premenstrual, give it a rub.

737 PAD IT OUT

If you're having problems with your lungs, chest area and breathing, give yourself a reflexology treatment by massaging the pad of the foot, under the toes as far down as the beginning of the arch.

738 PULL YOUR FINGER OUT

For some hand reflexology, grasp each finger or thumb at its base and tug firmly. Allow your grip to loosen slightly and let your finger gradually slide out of its grasp.

739 CENTRE YOURSELF

If you're feeling low or out of sorts, sit cross-legged or with knees dropped to the side on the floor with your thumbs gently pressing into the soles of your feet. This will help redress energy imbalance.

740 PINCH AN INCH

For headaches and stomach aches, pinch the webbing between the thumb and index finger and keep holding with the same pressure for a few minutes, when symptoms should start to disappear.

741 HEAD, FINGERS AND TOES

If you suffer from headaches, massaging toes and fingers could help reduce symptoms. Massage all fingers in turn but concentrate on the thumb and big toe.

742 REACH OUT

If you don't like your feet being touched but want to benefit from the relaxing effects of reflexology, try hand reflexology, which is based on the same principle but using hands instead of feet.

743 GET BACK IN LINE

To help reduce back pain, apply pressure with your thumb along the inside of each foot, starting at the base of the big toe and ending at the heel. Do this about ten times and gently massage any tender spots.

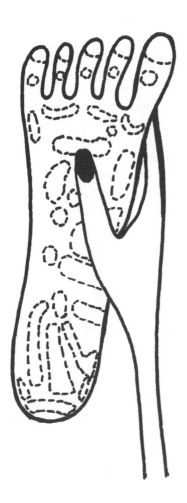

744 RUB IT OUT

To help relieve the symptoms of a cold, rub the balls of your feet with steady pressure. You can do the same to the pads under your fingers, but feet are more effective as there is more padding.

745 BE IMMUNE

Encourage strong immunity by massaging the reflexology points on the top of the foot between the toe and ankle with gentle pressure from the fingertips.

746 GIVE FINGERS A LIFT

For a quick hand boost, pinch the tops and bottoms of finger and thumb tips, then squeeze from side to side. They might feel a little uncomfortable, but you should never press if they are tender.

747 PALM IT OFF

Rest the palm of your hand inside your other palm and use your thumb to massage the back of your hand, starting with the knuckles and areas in between the knuckles and ending up near the wrist.

748 PRESS YOUR PALM

For a quick reflexology trick to help you centre your energy, relieve stress and encourage your body to take a few moments out, close your eyes, breathe deeply and press your thumb into the centre of your opposite palm for 30 seconds to a minute. Afterwards, open your eyes and rotate wrists to bring back energy.

749 SAY I LOVE YOU

If your child suffers from digestive complaints or constipation, give him or her an 'I Love You' double foot massage by using a thumb to trace an I (from the heel to the middle of their right foot), an L (across the feet in a line) and a U (in a line over the outside of the left foot, ending at the heel).

750 HEAL WITH REFLEXOLOGY

Although reflexology is not a substitute for a medical diagnosis, it can alleviate the symptoms of many health complaints, from migraines and PMS to back pain and poor digestion. It can kickstart the body into healing itself and strengthen immunity.

751 HAVE A BALL

If your thumbs and fingers get tired from massaging your feet, or you find the position uncomfortable, invest in some foot balls which you can use while sitting down to target treatment areas more comfortably.

752 GET SOME SOLE

A foot rub to the centre of the sole is a great way to help reduce the effects of a hangover, boost a detox or give you a lift if you're feeling down.

753 TWIST YOUR WRIST

A great self-massage for anyone who uses a computer or writes a lot is to massage the inside of your wrist with the thumb of the opposite hand. Move the wrist and hand around during the massage for greater effect.

754 GO GOLFING

To help give your feet a complete reflexology boost that will kickstart sluggish internal systems, stand on golf balls. It might sound painful but in fact it will give you a great energy boost.

neuro-linguistic programming (NLP)

755 PICTURE ACTIVITY

Exercise is a key factor in losing weight but many of us don't enjoy it. Trick your mind into enjoyment by picturing the times in your life when you enjoyed an activity (like sex or dancing). After a while, your unconscious mind will connect the feeling of excitement and eagerness to the thought of exercising.

756 FIGHT PHOBIAS

For phobias, NLP, which helps you 'rewire' your brain, can be a fantastic and relatively easy treatment. NLP claims to remove phobias in a couple of hours simply by altering your 'self-talk', the inner voice inside, replacing negative messages with positive ones.

757 VISUAL GOALS

Changes are implemented visually, auditorily and kinetically for greatest benefits in NLP, which means you need to see, hear and do them. Write down your goals and pin them to your fridge so you can see them, tell your family and friends what you're trying to do and put your plans into action.

758 REDUCE APPETITE WITH NLP

One of the basic NLP premises is that the mind and the body are one system. If you make a change in your mind, there will also be a change in the body. NLP can help reduce your appetite by helping you understand your eating habits. Create a mental picture of the times you snack and replace it with one of drinking water, walking or doing something healthy.

teenagers

759 GET A MENTOR

Your teenage years are really important in shaping what kind of adult you are going to become. Identify an adult you can treat as a mentor or role model in your life and go to for advice.

760 BURN THE CANDLE

Studies have shown that teenagers actually have different body clocks to people of other ages, being pre-programmed to stay up later and get up later too, so make sure you get enough rest if you want to be able to concentrate at school or college. Aim for eight or nine hours a night.

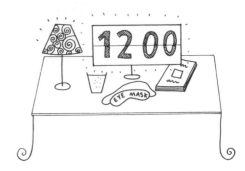

761 BE POSITIVE

It's really easy as a teenager to assume the world doesn't understand you, but take a minute to think about things from another point of view. Every time you feel angry at someone, try to think something positive about them.

762 ONLINE IS EASIER

You don't have to meet people face to face to discuss things. Many teenagers find talking about their feelings and emotions easier in online chat rooms where they can be anonymous.

763 CHOOSE YOUR ACTIVITIES

Instead of going along with friends who choose to do things you either don't like or aren't good at, try to opt for activities you enjoy and are good at as this will boost your self-esteem. Getting deeply involved in an activity, such as painting, dancing or music, can be therapeutic as well as satisfying.

764 BLOG IT

Create your own blog where you can work through thoughts and feelings as well as improving your communication skills. It might help you see problems differently and come up with solutions.

765 BE SAFE

If you go online, make sure you are careful about what information you give. Online predators are a reality so take care if someone asks for personal information and never meet an online friend alone.

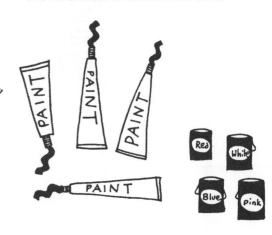

766 UNDERSTANDING DIVORCE

Lots of teenagers have to deal with their parents divorcing, but rest assured it's not your fault and it doesn't mean your parents don't love you. It can be a traumatic time, but being honest with both parents will help.

767 TALK IT THROUGH

Anger and resentment at a situation you can't control, like your parents splitting up, can cause you to feel frustrated with the rest of your life and even to start pushing friends away. Try to face up to your feelings rather than bottling them up. Find a friend or relative you can talk to – it can be a great release to get it off your chest.

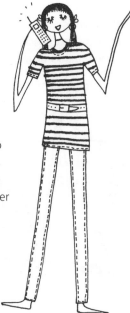

768 STI ALERT

Many teenagers feel they're invincible but when it comes to sexually transmitted infections, it really could be you. If you think something is wrong, see your doctor or clinic immediately.

769 STAY HYDRATED

Teenagers are prone to dehydration and it can affect not only your energy levels but also your ability to hit the books. Make sure you drink lots of water or clear fluids, and try to cut back on tea, coffee and fizzy drinks.

770 USE YOUR HEAD

Don't forget that your mental health is just as important as your physical health so aim to spend as much time looking after your mind as you do your body.

771 COVER UP

When it comes to STIs, condoms are really the only form of contraception that will give you protection. And if you have unprotected sex, don't forget it's like sleeping with everyone your partner has ever slept with.

772 KEEP IT QUIET

If your parents don't know you're sexually active, don't let that stop you seeking advice on sexual health. Everyone has the right to confidential treatment and it's important to get checked out.

773 BALANCE RESPONSIBILITIES

Being a teenager is tough – you're almost an adult but often parents won't give you the freedom you desire. Try to make a deal with them that meets them halfway to prove to them that you can take responsibility.

774 CHOOSE FOR YOURSELF

Don't let other people pressure you into making career or life decisions because of what they expect. Look at your strengths, weaknesses and desires, and choose a life path accordingly.

775 STAY TRUE TO YOURSELF

For teenagers embarking on their first romances, it can be hard to say no to sexual requests. Never do anything you don't feel comfortable with until you're ready.

776 YOU'RE NOT THE ONLY ONE

When chatting to your mates about sex and experience, remember that not everybody tells the truth when it comes to sex. In fact, most teenagers don't; chances are that they're just as confused as you are.

777 DON'T PILE ON THE PRESSURE

Be realistic about what you can expect from your exam results. Not everyone can get top grades or make it into the university of their choice, but everyone can do the best they can, so make that your goal.

778 TAKE YOUR TIME

Once the law says you're ready for adulthood it might be tempting to go all out and do as much as you can, but there's no rule saying that you have to be super-independent. Give yourself a little time to adjust to coming of age.

779 NO NEED FOR DIRECTION

There's increasing pressure on young people to know exactly what they want to do for the rest of their lives. Don't pressure yourself to choose a career too early if you're not sure; just keep your options open.

780 ONE STEP AT A TIME

Don't forget that your parents have looked after you since you were a tiny baby, so it's no surprise that your newfound independence can be difficult for them. Try taking small steps towards it rather than jumping away from them.

781 GET ACTIVE

With so many other distractions, many teenagers stop exercising but studies show it's important to keep active, not only to help your body stay strong (because it's still developing) but to boost concentration, too.

782 THINK AHEAD

If you're not sure about career or college choices, don't stress about it by yourself; open up to someone you trust and talk about what's worrying you. Friends may brag they know exactly what they want to do, but they might not be being honest.

twenties

783 BE SAFE

The top three causes of death for people in their twenties are accidents, especially car accidents, murder and suicide. Help reduce your risk by being vigilant about your personal safety and avoiding dangerous situations.

784 MAKE FRIENDS

Studies have also shown that people with a strong friendship network live longer and healthier lives, and it's the friends you make in your twenties who stay around forever, so make time to get out there and meet people.

785 QUIT THE WEED

Nothing takes years off your life faster than smoking, and while the risks to your health aren't enormous in your twenties, you're setting yourself up for problems in years to come. Now is the time to quit.

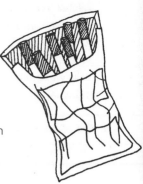

786 DON'T OVERDO IT

The twenties is the time when you have most energy and are fittest, but make sure you avoid over-exercising. This can not only lead to injury, but can actually have detrimental effects on your body's internal systems like liver and digestion. If in doubt, ask for advice.

787 START LIFTING WEIGHTS

Although your body doesn't start to gradually lose muscle mass until you're in your thirties, it's important to start lifting weights in your twenties in order to help your muscles stay strong for longer.

788 KNOW YOUR NEEDS

Your twenties are a great time to learn how to deal with relationships – both with partners and friends – to work out what you really want from your nearest and dearest and what they need from you in return.

789 EXERCISE FOR THE FUTURE

Use your twenties – when other responsibilities are likely to be fewer – to establish an exercise routine you can keep up as you get older. Work out what activities you like and get a routine that fits your lifestyle. The physical decline that doesn't usually start until you reach your thirties or forties can start in the twenties for people who shun exercise.

790 BE POSITIVE

Studies show that having a positive perception about ageing can add as much as seven years to your life. Ageing is not an inevitable decline in function and ability and if you adopt healthy behaviours while you are young, you can have a healthy long life.

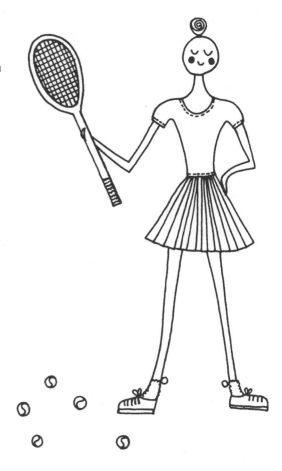

thirties

791 WORK AT IT

It is estimated that a quarter of thirty-somethings in relationships are unhappy with the state of the relationship. If you feel your relationship needs a boost, talk to your partner and seek professional help if necessary.

792 THE FAMILY TRAP

One of the reasons people stay in failing relationships in their thirties is that they are worried time is running out for raising a family. Remember that any relationship weaknesses will be magnified by having children, and many couples aren't starting their families until later these days.

793 DON'T HOLD BACK

Research has shown that almost a quarter of people in their thirties who want to change career don't because of a lack of confidence. Your thirties are a great time to make changes, so grab the chance with both hands.

794 AVOID A CRISIS

Forget mid-life crises, there's a growing phenomenon of crises in people in their thirties. Remember the three Fs – fun, fulfilment and freedom.

795 HAVE SEX

Self-esteem and body image is better in people over 30 who have sex – they are likely to have greater emotional wellbeing, especially in long-term relationships, which foster togetherness.

796 DITCH THE BAGGAGE

If you're carrying around old resentments and issues from earlier in your life, which are having a negative impact on your life now, deal with them once and for all. If necessary, seek professional help.

797 BE GOOD TO YOURSELF

Your thirties are often filled with family responsibilities and long working hours, but don't neglect your own health as this is the decade that age-related health problems can start to occur.

798 BOOST YOUR CONFIDENCE

Surveys have shown that three-quarters of people in their thirties wish they were more confident. Hold a confidence-boosting evening with your friends where you tell each other your best characteristics.

799 KNOW YOUR CORE VALUES

By the time you reach your thirties, chances are you will know what's really valuable to you. Understanding what's most important to you in life enables you to prioritize.

800 THROW AWAY THE SCRIPT

All of us have certain roles – at work, home, with family and friends. Your thirties is the time to realize what boxes you fit into in your relationships and start to get rid of roles you're not comfortable with.

801 TAKE A LONG VIEW

By the time you've reached your thirties, it's likely that you'll have decided upon a career. To avoid your life becoming narrowly focused, create a 'big vision' to give yourself a sense of direction and purpose.

802 TAKE RESPONSIBILITY

If you're still relying on other people to get you through life, or blaming them for your problems, your thirties is the time to finally take responsibility and become accountable for what goes on in your life.

forties

803 HORMONE PILL

Your body's levels of progesterone begin to decline in preparation for menopause, which can cause increased pre-menstrual symptoms. Hormone pills are effective, so seek help if your periods suddenly become worse.

804 SPOT STRESS

It's not just teenagers who suffer from acne – if you find your skin becomes prone to breakouts in your forties it's most likely because of stress. Learning some breathing techniques, meditation or exercising can all help treat the root cause.

805 BEAR SOME WEIGHT

Women and, to a lesser extent, men become increasingly susceptible to the bone-wasting disease osteoporosis in their forties. Weight-bearing exercise such as free weights, running and yoga can help counteract the effects of ageing.

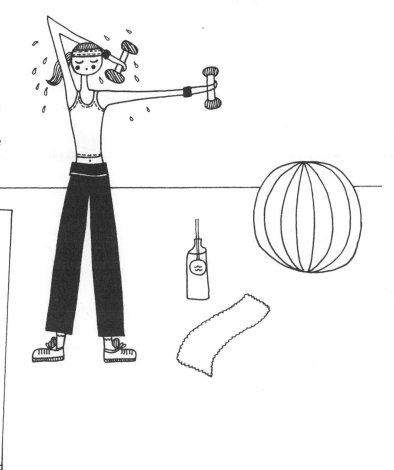

806 LOOK AFTER MUSCLES

More time needs to be spent warming up and cooling down before exercise in your forties, as muscles are weaker and more prone to strain. Aim for 5–10 minutes before and 10–20 after.

807 TAKE A LOAD OFF

Almost a third of forty-somethings work full time and most are still working long hours, with many citing 'too heavy a work load' as one of the major causes of stress in their life. Talk to your managers if it's problematic.

808 DITCH THE YO-YO

If you've been a yo-yo dieter in your life, your forties is the time to take extra care with your vitamin intake as the regular periods of 'starvation' your body has undergone may have had a lasting effect on metabolism.

809 MINERAL RICH

People in their forties should aim for a diet rich in iron, magnesium, calcium and zinc, all of which can help your body fight the signs and symptoms of ageing.

810 BE SUPPORTIVE

By the time you reach your forties the chances are you've started – or are about to start – experiencing problems with ageing parents, which can be a significant source of stress. Discuss responsibilities with siblings beforehand to help reduce the load.

811 MAKE YOURSELF HAPPY

Research shows that people in their forties are more stressed than any other age group, so it's even more important to take action to reduce stress, like making sure you have quality time alone and with your loved ones, doing things that make you happy.

812 DON'T DIET

Habitual dieters who snack on high-sugar foods when hungry tend to have a higher blood-sugar level than others, which the body deals with by drawing calcium from the bones. Make sure your calcium intake is high and take supplements if necessary, to avoid osteoporosis.

813 **CUT THE CARBS**

In your forties, cut down on simple carbohydrates such as bread, pasta and potatoes in favour of fresh fruit and vegetables that contain the minerals and nutrients needed for a healthy body, particularly calcium.

fifties

814 **GET ACTIVE**

The best cure for the blues is activity. Get some friends together for a walk, join a walking or garden-visiting group or simply get out in your own garden.

815 **NO NEED TO WIND DOWN**

Instead of seeing your fifties as a time for winding down and preparing for getting older, try to see it as a time of personal opportunity where you know yourself well and have time to enjoy life. Take the time to organize travel or social activities that keep you having new experiences.

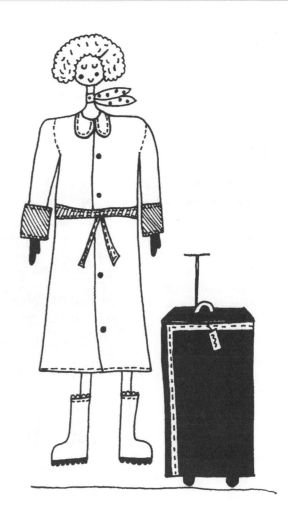

816 HAVE A DAILY PLAN

Don't put off until tomorrow what you can do today. Many people say what helps them to feel good is waking up in the morning and knowing what is planned for the day.

817 DON'T BE RIGID

One of the best ways to stay positive is to have a day plan (see above), but don't let your plans rule you – variety is the spice of life so if an unexpected offer comes up or it's sunny and you want to get outside, don't be afraid to ditch the plan.

818 MAKE A LIFESTYLE CHOICE

As you get older, it's even more important to start making choices that impact on your life. For instance, why not save the money you normally spend on taxis, cigarettes or wine? Then you can use the extra money to get something that will make a real difference to your life – like a cleaner!

819 GIVE SOME CARE

Most women, and many men, in their fifties take on a caring role for family members but be careful not to let this define you. Make sure you carve out time for yourself as well as helping others.

820 BALANCE YOUR MONEY

The basic rule to keep in mind in your fifties when you're planning for your financial future is that you don't want to run out of money before you run out of years.

821 ENJOY IT

Medical researchers have established that women may derive more pleasure from sex as they grow older because they no longer have anxieties about contraception, but you should still use condoms if you're sleeping with someone new to protect against disease.

822 SPEAK OUT

Many people feel they become invisible as they age and are too afraid to speak out against discrimination. Make it a rule to challenge discrimination if it happens to you.

823 BALANCE IT OUT

Reduced activity naturally leads to reduced balance. Keep yours in tune with martial arts like tai chi or yoga, which will keep you strong and supple as well as in balance.

824 EARLY SIGNS

Your fifties is when the first signs of many diseases like heart disease and cancers start to appear. It's the best time to start medical screening so you can catch problems early.

825 REDEFINE YOUR TERMS

Instead of thinking of 'ageing' as a mental and physical deterioration (the most common reaction), try to think of it positively. Use words like 'maturing' if 'ageing' frightens you.

826 GET MENTALLY EMPOWERED

If you are worried about becoming forgetful or losing your mental sharpness, try a supplement formulated for the over-fifties that boosts mental agility. These usually contain a cocktail of B-complex vitamins, omega 3 and omega 6 fatty acids, ginkgo biloba and taurine.

827 CHANGE THINGS AROUND

Women over 50 are actually more likely to have a higher sex drive than men, with sex being more important to them than their partners. Keep him interested by not sticking to the same old routine. Sex is also more closely linked to wellbeing for people in their fifties than for any other age group.

828 BEAR WEIGHT FOR GOOD BONES

It's really important to make sure at least one of your weekly activities is load-bearing, like running, lifting weights or yoga, as this will help prevent osteoporosis. Make sure you are tested regularly for bone density, too, and follow any advice if a problem is found. The earlier it's detected, the better the results with treatment.

829 GET SOME CALCIUM

Losing bone mass is a problem widely experienced by older women, but making sure you have enough calcium in your fifties could help your bones stay stronger for longer. Take a supplement and eat dairy produce, green vegetables and fish.

830 CUT OUT SODIUM

Everyone in their fifties should watch their intake of high-sodium foods and fizzy drinks, which can reduce bone mass.

831 CONSIDER DOWNSIZING

By your fifties, it's likely that your home has a lot of equity so it may be time to think about downsizing, which will free up some money to make your retirement years more comfortable.

832 TWEAK YOUR MONEY

If you have planned well financially for your old age, don't rest on your laurels. Instead, make sure you pay regular attention to your finances and work out the best way to make them work for you.

833 PLAN AHEAD

The whole attitude behind financial planning begins to change by the time you reach your fifties. Ten years earlier, retirement seemed very far away but now it seems imminent. Start thinking long-term now if you haven't already.

834 START NOW

Instead of waiting until you're older to think about how to stay happy and healthy, start now – it's a great time to join bridge or social clubs that will help you develop a long-lasting network of friends.

835 SWAP TO GENTLER SPORTS

If you're quite active you may need to slow the pace slightly. Golf, tennis and swimming can see you into an active old age.

836 RECONSIDER INSURANCE

When you had a growing family, your life insurance requirements were large but you may be able to cut your insurance and switch the premiums to investments. Talk to an independent financial advisor.

837 SHIFT YOUR SAVINGS

While you may have been bold with your savings and investments when you were younger, now is not the time to take risks. Switch savings to less volatile investments like bonds, but avoid putting all your eggs in one basket.

sixties

838 FIGHT ALZHEIMER'S

Vitamins C and E are thought to help lower the risk of Alzheimer's disease, and making sure your fresh foods are of good quality and eating them in raw or lightly cooked form rather than overcooked maximizes health giving effects.

839 WATCH THE SUGAR

As you get older, your body is more prone to sugar highs and lows and less able to deal with high-sugar foods. It's important to include lots of fibre and wholegrain in your diet.

840 DRINK UP

Older people are more prone to dehydration and should drink more water than when they were younger, not less. Drinking at least eight glasses a day will help to keep your body organs functioning optimally and keep skin looking younger as well.

841 TRY SOMETHING NEW

It's never too late to be a student, so make it a rule to learn something new every day. Even if it's something you read in the paper or hear on the news, making an effort to retain new information will help keep your brain feeling young.

842 TAKE A BREAK

Many retired people find volunteering is a great way to meet new people and keep themselves busy. But if you volunteer, make sure you don't work yourself into the ground – take regular breaks and ask for help if you need it.

843 GET A COMPANION

If you are living on your own, consider getting a pet. A cat is a good low-maintenance pet but if you are active, consider a dog. Older pets have less energy, which means they are not nearly as demanding as younger animals. They will provide companionship and give you a sense of purpose.

844 EAT UP

In your sixties, your appetite begins to wane and foods seem less appealing as your metabolism slows down. Staying active can help limit this decline so that you won't gain weight even with a little extra food.

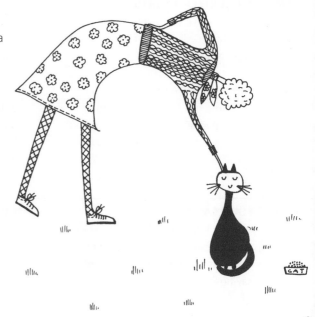

845 IF YOU DON'T USE IT, YOU LOSE IT

Your taste buds will be less sharp at 60 than they used to be, but to keep them going strong for as long as possible it's important to keep trying different foods and tastes.

846 EAT OFTEN

Because your appetite is likely to have reduced, even if you are still active, it might be easier to eat four or five smaller meals a day, rather than three large ones, to help keep your blood sugar levels constant.

847 DON'T SLOW DOWN

Don't think that because you are in your sixties you have to slow down your activity to a gentler pace – as long as you are healthy, vigorous exercise is a great way to keep your body looking and feeling young.

848 THINK WHOLEGRAIN

Make sure you include wholegrains like barley, brown rice, wholemeal bread and quinoa in your diet because they contain lots of fibre which will help keep your digestive tract in top form.

849 TAKE A PROBIOTIC

About 90% of the bacteria in the gut of a newborn infant are 'friendly', but this drops to 10–15% in the average adult and after the age of 60, they could be a thousand times less. Taking a probiotic could help.

850 MOISTURIZE

Your skin will now be telling the effects of how well you looked after it in previous decades, but all post-menopausal women need to moisturize as the lack of oestrogen means the skin is dryer.

851 AVOID THE SUN

In your sixties, pigmentation marks can start to show, with some areas being lighter or darker than others, sometimes in large patches. It's best to avoid the sun altogether, or make sure you're covered up with an spf 30+ sunscreen.

852 JOIN A GYM

Keeping going when your body is weaker may require more willpower. Joining a gym can help not only with programmes but also with a social scene to help you stay focused.

853 KEEP UP THE ACTIVITY

The levels of DHEA growth hormone drop dramatically by the time you reach your sixties, meaning keeping muscle is harder. Sixty-somethings who don't exercise are ill more often, lose more mobility, have more trouble sleeping and lose coordination much more quickly – so get active.

854 WEIGHT LIFT

Lifting weights, or other load-bearing exercise like running and team sports, helps put a stop to muscle wastage and bone density decline, which is especially important for post-menopausal women.

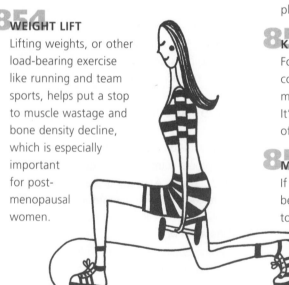

seventies

855 BE SAFE AT HOME

As you get older you are more prone to falls and accidents, so take a few minutes to check your home for possible hazards, such as dimly lit stairs and hallways. Also avoid standing on chairs and stools to reach high places or light bulbs.

856 KEEP FEET HEALTHY

Foot pain and other problems with feet can contribute to an increased risk of falls so make sure you see a chiropodist regularly. It's also important to wear the correct type of shoes as you get older.

857 MAKE A CALL

If someone comes to your door claiming to be from a utilities company, don't be afraid to make a call to that company to check their ID. Make sure you get the number from a separate source, like your own bill or directory – genuine callers will not mind waiting.

858 IT'S A BALANCING ACT

Exercising regularly, particularly making sure that you concentrate on types of activity which help balance and strength like pilates, tai chi and yoga, is the best defence against falls.

859 DON'T BE DIZZY

Some medicines can make you dizzy and increase your risk of falling and hurting yourself. If you suffer dizziness as a side effect of your medication, talk to your doctor for advice.

860 GET AN EYE TEST

Have your eyes tested regularly. Not only is it important to get your eyes checked so that you are not straining them and causing further damage, eye tests can also help pick up on other problems such as diabetes.

861 FRESH AIR FOR EYES

When our bodies come into contact with natural sunlight they are stimulated to produce vitamin D, which helps keep bones healthy and strong. Aim for half an hour of fresh air a day.

862 AVOID LARGE BILLS

The aim with all your spending should be to spread bill payments over the year so that your outgoings match your income in amount and frequency.

863 KNOW THE SIGNS OF DEHYDRATION

If you're suffering from any of the following, drink fluids immediately: thirst, dry mouth and skin, or cracked lips; dark-coloured urine; feeling tired, confused or having a headache.

864 SEE YOUR DOCTOR

You should always see a doctor for an assessment following a fall, even if you don't think you were badly hurt. If you have regular falls, they can help by running a falls risk assessment.

865 USE RESEARCH

If you have to buy something new and aren't sure you're being sold the right thing, seek independent advice from a consumer protection association that will give impartial advice first.

866 DON'T KEEP CASH

One of the reasons criminals target older people in their homes is because they are likely to keep cash in large amounts. Keep your money in a bank or at the post office instead for safety and peace of mind.

867 COMPARE QUOTES

When you need to have work done, get at least two or three separate quotes from different tradespeople, and don't be pressured into parting with money in advance.

868 A RAINY DAY ACCOUNT

If you want to save regularly for vacations, celebrations or unexpectedly large bills, get a savings account with a bank, but remember these accounts often have notice periods for withdrawals.

869 CHECK YOUR HOME

Don't wait until your appliances and household items break before thinking about replacing or repairing them. Check them regularly and keep abreast of sales and offers so you don't have to panic buy.

870 GET UP SOON

If you do fall and aren't too badly hurt, get up as soon as you can because a lot of the problems people experience after falls are from lying on the ground for too long and getting cold. Pull or push yourself up if possible.

over-eighties

871 KEEP MOVING

Studies have shown that 'exercise deficiency syndrome' is the biggest risk to older people. Regular exercise prevents high blood pressure, heart disease, stroke, poor circulation, depression, obesity, and joint and bone problems.

872 BE A SOCIALITE

Having a strong network of family and friends and a range of activities is vital to the health of your mind and body, not only because it makes you feel happier, but because mental stimulation is important to stay alert and engaged with life.

873 SEEK HELP

Don't put up with health problems on the grounds of 'age' or assume that old age means nothing can be done. Age is not a cause of illness, and it is not a reason for sub-standard healthcare, either.

874 STAY HYDRATED

Remember that alcohol and caffeine are diuretics. Although you still take in more liquid than you lose from a cup of tea, coffee or a cola-type soft drink, you should try to balance them with clear fluids. Make it a rule of thumb to carry a bottle of water with you everywhere in the summer, so you make absolutely sure you don't get dehydrated.

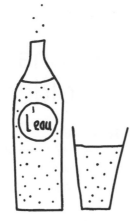

875 LITTLE AND OFTEN

People who regularly drink small amounts of alcohol tend to live longer than people who don't drink at all because alcohol helps prevent coronary heart disease. The maximum benefit is achieved by drinking between one and two units of alcohol a day.

876 THINK POSITIVE

Every day, spend 20 minutes focused on a really uplifting thought or memory – you will feel better and your immune system will get a boost. Be positive about your wants and needs too – studies show that longevity appears to be linked to a determination to stay in control.

877 MENTAL AGILITY

Research shows that cognitive functions can be kept agile by doing regular mental gymnastics. Crosswords, Sudoku and puzzles are excellent mental gyms, as are discussion groups and many kinds of voluntary work.

878 BE ASPIRING

Talk to your doctor about taking aspirin regularly. There is some evidence that it can help to prevent coronary thrombosis, cancer of the colon and possibly cataracts. Not everyone can tolerate aspirin so it's important to check with your doctor, especially if you have gastric problems.

879 COVER UP TO STAY WARM

It seems obvious, but putting on an extra layer or wrapping up under a blanket can keep you warm if your home is cold, especially at night. Keep a blanket near your bed for the early hours and wear layers – several layers are much easier to adjust than a heavy jumper (sweater).

880 GET GREAT GUMS

Gum disease is often the cause of lost teeth, so brush your gums gently and see the dentist if they bleed. If you wear dentures, make sure they fit properly; dentures need to be changed from time to time as your jaw changes shape with age.

881 BRUSH AWAY

Older adults are likely to take medications that can impact oral health. And as you get older, dental health is more important because loose and missing teeth can cause problems eating, which can lead to malnutrition. Brush twice a day and get regular check-ups from a dentist.

882 THE EYES HAVE IT

Eating foods rich in lutein – such as sweetcorn, spinach, courgettes, green peppers, cucumbers, red grapes and kiwis – is thought to help protect against cataracts and macular degeneration.

seasonal changes for older people

883 GET A JAB

Everyone over 70 should get a flu jab every year to help protect them against the likely strains of flu, which can be dangerous in older people.

884 MOVE FOR WARMTH

In the winter, many old people get dangerously cold because they don't move around. Even vacuuming or doing some gentle exercise in the home can help get circulation moving again.

885 TOP UP YOUR POTASSIUM

Fruit and vegetables are not only good to include in your diet because of their mineral and vitamin content, the potassium they contain is also thought to increase sodium (salt) excretion. Potassium is found in meat, bananas, dried fruits, potatoes and avocado.

886 STAY IN MIDDAY

Avoid going out during the hottest part of the day in the summer, which is from about 11 am to about 3 pm. If you have to go out during this time, stay in the shade, wear a hat and loose-fitting clothes and make sure your shoes are sensible. The idea is to stay as cool as possible, so natural fabrics are best.

887 INSULATE IN THE SUMMER

Double glazing, loft and cavity wall insulation are good for summer as well as winter. Use draught-proofing strips and thick curtains in the winter.

888 KEEP WARM AT NIGHT

Keep your window closed, and help your health too – cold air on the head at night has been shown to raise blood pressure in older people, so stay warm if you can.

889 START EARLY

If you want to spend some time in your garden in the summer, try to do it early in the morning or in the evening as the sun is going down, which means you'll be able to relax rather than overheat.

890 EAT FOR TEMPERATURE

In the winter, two or three hot meals a day and regular hot drinks provide warmth and energy, and in the summer remember to drink lots of cool water and juices, and eat fruit and cold meals.

becoming a grandparent

891 SHARE EXPECTATIONS

You're bound to be excited about the prospect of becoming a grandparent, but don't assume your children will know what you want from it – talk to them about your expectations and theirs so you all know what to expect.

892 HOLD BACK

There's nothing guaranteed to ruin the joy of being a new parent more than a grandparent interfering and constantly talking about how things used to be. Bite your tongue and let your children do it their way.

893 BE PREPARED

Instead of relying on your children to fill you in on the dizzying array of new technology around childbirth, why not do some research yourself so you will know what to expect. The internet, doctors and libraries are all good sources.

894 ASK QUESTIONS

Don't be afraid to ask your children whether they are planning a family of their own. If you are open to their answers and not judgemental, they will relish the chance to talk about their decisions.

895 TAKE A CLASS

Many hospitals and groups run classes for grandparents-to-be, helping fill you in on the nitty-gritty of what to expect as well as explaining the methods and techniques that have changed since your day.

896 OFFER SUPPORT

Remember that your job as a grandparent is not only to support your new grandchild but also your children – they are likely to need you a lot more after the birth than they have for several years.

897 START EARLY

Don't assume your job starts when the baby is born – the last few months of a pregnancy are a great time to start bonding and laying the foundations for a good relationship.

898 BE ADAPTABLE

It's good to start talking as early as possible about what your input as a grandparent will be – will it be daycare, babysitting or maybe financial? But don't set anything in stone; all of you may change your mind once the baby comes along.

899 WAIT TILL YOU'RE ASKED

Your children know you have lots of advice and experience to give, but don't risk ruining your relationship by offering it unless they ask. Try to express doubts or worries in non-threatening ways and always be ready to listen – your children may need someone to unload their worries to but that doesn't mean they will necessarily take any advice you offer.

900 STAY YOUNG

Being a grandparent should be fun – free of responsibility and full of laughter – all the benefits without the burdens. If you find your 'job' of caring for your grand-children is making you feel older rather than younger, maybe it's time to put limits in place.

901 ENJOY THE SPOILS

Many grandparents look forward to spoiling their grandchildren, but make sure this means lots of love and time rather than disregarding their parents' rules or giving them everything they ask for.

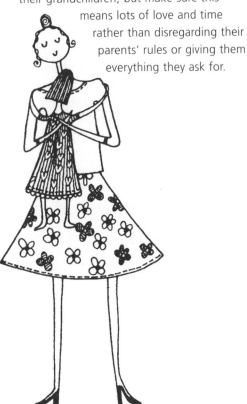

age discrimination

902 OMIT DATES

When applying for a new job, leave out any dates that will age you from your covering letter and CV (résumé). Put the focus on your recent job experience and keep it to the last 10–15 years and to relevant jobs.

903 GAIN NEW SKILLS

If you're looking for a new job, try spending some time updating your skills. Employers respond well to people who adapt to change, and learning new skills is a great way to demonstrate flexibility.

904 POSITIVE ATTITUDE

Don't go about looking for work thinking people don't want you because you're older. Negativity is catching, so work at projecting a positive image which is bright, neat and alert, and concentrate on what you can offer TODAY, in addition to your wealth of experience.

905 EMBRACE CHANGE

Be adaptable in your approach to finding new work and embrace new opportunities and responsibilities. If you are forward-thinking enough, prospective employers won't notice your age.

being a student

906 HEAD DOWN

Studying at home can be tough, as the rest of the family often don't understand how to help, or want to. Try to talk to them reasonably about what would help you in the run-up to exams and ask them what you could do for them in return when your exams are over.

907 BE SURE TO ASK

Often, a cause of people failing at school is not understanding what's needed when it comes to homework or assignments. Talk to your teacher or lecturer and make sure you know exactly what's required.

908 KEEP IT VARIED

University is an opportunity to learn about life as well as your chosen subject so make sure you don't just stick to the course. Check out public noticeboards for groups or clubs and join a few to further your interests.

909 EAT BREAKFAST

Even if you're getting up halfway through the day, eating breakfast is an essential way to start your day. When it comes to keeping your energy high for studying, it's even more important.

910 GET REGISTERED

It's important to make sure you register with a local doctor or clinic as soon if you have travelled to study in a new town so that you can seek help quickly and easily if you become ill.

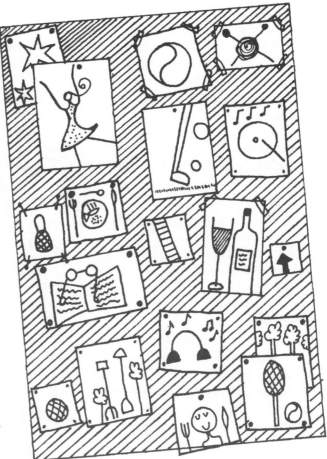

911 PLAN THE REST

In the run-up to exams, try to give your memory a break by writing down to-do lists and work plans, both for revision and after the exam period, rather than keeping them in your head. It will help focus your time-keeping as well.

912 TAKE AN HOUR

For one hour a day, do something that has nothing to do with your course. Watching TV or doing an exercise class can help clear your mind, or simply have a coffee break or take a walk with your friends.

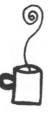

913 DO IT HOURLY

Split each hour you spend studying into work time and break time to make sure you're working most effectively. Work for 45–50 minutes and then take a 10–15 minute break, which will leave you refreshed for the next stint. Working without breaks is non-productive.

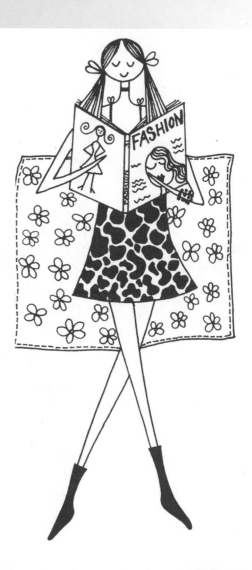

914 GET PHYSICAL

Take care of your physical health by exercising at least three times a week. You may never have as many opportunities to join sports teams and clubs again, so there's no excuse. A tennis match or a few laps in the pool are great ways to relieve tension too.

915 KEEP YOUR FRIENDS

Even if your course is ultra-demanding, make sure you don't isolate yourself at university or college. Making time for your friends is really important, as they will help reduce your stress.

916 HAVE FUN

Studying can be a lonely business. Make a point to schedule some fun into your day. For instance, make a rule that you won't work after 9.30 pm and get out of the house to meet some friends.

917 SEEK ADVICE

If you do become ill while away from home and need to get some rest, make sure someone knows, so they can check on you – in case you worsen or get dehydrated.

918 KEEP UP-TO-DATE

Medical experts suggest that before you embark on your university or college career you make sure your vaccinations are up to date, especially for meningitis C, which is common among students.

919 TAKE A BREAK

When it comes to the breaks from college or university, lots of students need to work, but make sure you give yourself at least a few weeks a year when you take time out to relax and recharge.

920 GET A ROUTINE

Try to timetable your studying so you sit down in the same place at the same time each day. This will give your brain and body a chance to get used to studying and make you more efficient.

921 SET YOURSELF LIMITS

When it comes to exams, there will always be more to do than you can achieve, so don't get bogged down. Write your list in order of priority and set time limits for each item.

922 DON'T OVERDO IT

It's tempting to join in with everything you can when you first start college or university, but try to be realistic about what you can handle. Working and playing too hard and not getting enough rest can lead to anxiety and depression, so stay sensible.

923 MAKE A STUDY DATE

Don't always study alone when it comes to exam revision. Study with a friend but don't just stick to the same ones. For each subject, choose people of the same ability and who are compatible with your way of learning and form separate groups.

924 STAY AWAY

Resist the urge to go home every weekend. Leaving home for the first time can be a difficult adjustment, but you're likely to cope with it better and stop feeling homesick quicker if you throw yourself into your new surroundings and don't leave every week. It will also give you the opportunity to develop new friends, which can take time.

925 EAT REGULARLY

Skipping meals has been shown to lead to snacking on high-fat, high-calorie, sugary foods, which are not nutritious. Also, it has been scientifically proven that meal skippers accomplish less work, are physically unsteady and slower at making decisions. Avoid empty calories and feed your body and brain nutritiously on a regular basis.

926 GET A THIRD STARCH

For best energy levels, aim to make a third of your food starchy – for example, bread, pasta and rice. A great way of doing it is to mentally divide your plate into three and make sure a third is filled with starchy stuff.

927 SAY NO TO SUGAR

When you're studying until the early hours, snack on foods like cereal or sandwiches rather than high-sugar foods or drinks which can actually reduce concentration. Bear in mind that a can of coke contains 8 rounded teaspoons of sugar, a pack of boiled sweets (hard candy) 24 teaspoons and a typical chocolate bar 9.

928 FIVE-A-DAY

Make sure you take in at least five portions of fruit and vegetables a day, especially if you are hitting the town, to help make up for lack of sleep and increased alcohol intake. For student cooking, frozen vegetables are great choices.

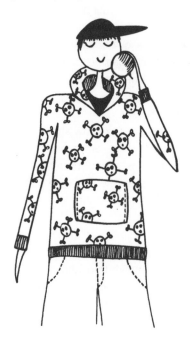

929 BE COMPLEMENTARY

For vegetarians, the best way to ensure you're getting enough protein is to eat foods in the right mixtures, like cereal foods with dairy or pulses, and pulses with seeds or nuts.

930 FEED YOUR BRAIN

Keep the brain well nourished with a diet rich in fish oils (omega 3 and 6), B-complex vitamins (in cereals and grains), folic acid (in fresh vegetables and fruits), zinc (in cereals and nuts) and vitamin A (in dark green leafy vegetables and orange or yellow fruits).

931 CARB HEAVY

If you're cooking on a budget, snack in between meals on starchy, simple foods such as cereal, toast or a baked potato, which will keep you going for a long time.

932 GET LEAN

Instead of buying large amounts of fatty meat of which you will have to waste lots, try buying a small amount of leaner meat like chicken or lean steak. You will be able to use more of it and it will be healthier.

933 FIND YOUR PULSE

Beans, peas and lentils are a cheap source of protein and are great for using to bulk up stews, soups and casseroles with, or instead of, meat. One-pot meals like casseroles are great because they can be used for more than one meal – and save on washing up!

934 COMMUNAL COOKING

If you live in a student house, instead of everyone cooking for themselves every night, create a cooking club where you take turns to cook for each other a few nights a week. It will give you a rest and help you socialize. It will also save you money in ingredients.

935 MARKET SAVVY

Instead of buying fruit and vegetables at a supermarket where they can be expensive and high on packaging, why not visit a market? Most towns and cities have one and students usually have some time off in the day to shop, so are well placed to find healthy bargains.

936 CAN IT

If you can't afford fresh fruit and vegetables, particularly if it's out of season, buy them canned in natural juice or water, which keep well.

937 CLUB TOGETHER

Instead of each buying your own meat source if you live in student accommodation, why not club together for a joint of meat to share and add your own accompaniments. Cheap joints like shoulders of lamb are great choices.

938 STOCK UP A STORE

At the beginning of term, buy store-cupboard essentials like lentils, beans, dry pasta, packet soups, peanut butter, canned fruit and vegetables. These will see you through when money is tight.

939 REHEAT WELL

When reheating food leftovers make sure everything is piping hot throughout, particularly if you're using a microwave, which can heat irregularly. Do it within 48 hours and don't reheat more than once.

pregnancy

940 PUT YOUR FEET UP

Feet and ankles can often get sore and swollen in pregnancy because of fluid retention and the added weight you're carrying around. Whenever you can, rest with your feet elevated to help fluid drainage.

941 GET COMFY

Sleeping on your left side with your knees slightly raised is often considered the best position for you and your baby because it is said to help relieve nausea as well as increase blood flow to the foetus and decrease swelling. Put a pillow between your legs for extra comfort.

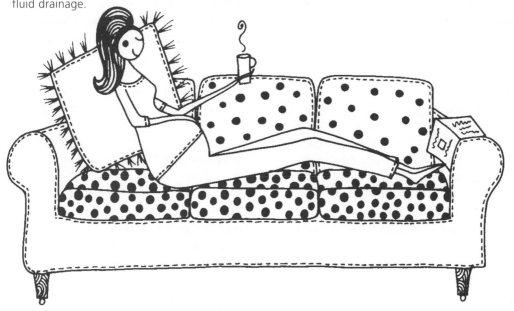

942 CONNECT WITH YOURSELF

Antenatal yoga is a great choice during pregnancy because it not only helps you stretch and relax hard-working muscles but it will also help you connect with the changes in your body.

943 BE POSITIVE

Being pregnant involves a lot of tests and information about things that could go wrong but bear in mind that most pregnancies are fine and try to focus on the positive.

944 JOIN A GROUP

Wherever you can, join groups that will help you meet women who are going through the same experience as you. Not only will making pregnant friends help you now, they'll be invaluable when your kids come along.

945 SPLASH ABOUT

Swimming is ideal exercise during pregnancy as your body is weightless, so reducing pressure on joints and muscles. The breaststroke and backstroke are the best strokes to use during pregnancy.

946 BODY AWARE

Skin, hair and nail growth often changes during pregnancy so make sure you alter the products you buy accordingly. Use a good moisturizer on your stomach and breasts to avoid stretch marks. Taking care of your body will make you feel nurtured.

947 SLEEP IT OUT

Night-time toilet visits become a frequent occurrence throughout pregnancy but to minimize them, avoid caffeinated foods and drinks, reduce the amount of fluids you consume in the hours before bedtime and take a trip to the toilet before you settle for the night.

948 STRETCH OUT CRAMPS

If you suffer from leg cramps during the night you should gently stretch the muscle and massage the area until the pain has subsided. Stretching out your calf muscles before bed may help to reduce their incidence, as will making sure you're properly hydrated – lack of fluids is one of the main causes of cramping.

949 DREAM EASY

Many women suffer from vivid dreams or nightmares during pregnancy, and the broken sleep patterns make it more likely you'll remember them. Try not to worry about dreams, but do talk to your partner or a friend if they are making you anxious.

950 ENJOY SOME ADULT TIME

Pregnancy is the last chance you'll have for a while to enjoy some time with your partner and friends, so make the most of it. Try to go on a date with your partner every few weeks to just enjoy being together.

951 TRAVEL SAFELY

If you're flying during pregnancy, make sure you wear support stockings. When you're pregnant your fluid levels increase and you're more prone to swollen feet and ankles.

952 SAY NO TO SPICE

To avoid night-time indigestions, avoid eating heavy or spicy meals before bed. Instead, snack on plain food such as a banana, toast or crackers, and drink milk or herbal tea.

parenting

953 ENCOURAGE PERSISTENCE

Don't teach children to be perfect; teach them to be persistent because that is what is more likely to bring them success in life. Going after perfection brings with it a fear of failure, which won't help their future.

954 A POSITIVE OUTLOOK

One of the biggest indicators of happiness in adults is how positive their outlook is and parents can help their children grow up positive by concentrating on the good – 'well done for cleaning your room'; 'don't forget to put your socks in the drawer' rather than, 'you haven't done it properly, your socks are still out'.

955 HELP THEM FOCUS

It's important to instil a sense of achievement into your children so they understand that effort and hard work are linked to praise and pleasure – adults who don't make this connection, end up by not achieving things.

956 MAKE SUNDAY SPECIAL

It has been shown that families who spend time together at weekends (or any other specified day if weekends are difficult for you) develop closer links and are less likely to suffer depression.

957 WRITE A LIST

If your child is resistant to school, get them to write a list of everything they like and don't like about school and work with them to reduce the 'don't like' list. Enlist the help of their teacher if necessary.

958 LOOK AFTER YOURSELF

Research shows that the number-one worry for children is the health of a loved one. Children count on their families so make sure you give the right message by showing them you look after your health.

959 TALK IT THROUGH

Talk to your children rather than shouting at them. If they have done something wrong, explain what it was rather than expecting them to read your mind. Keep your thoughts positive and it will rub off on them.

960 TEACH THEM WELL

Remember that today's children are tomorrow's adults, and it falls to you to help them develop the capacity for happiness. Each day when you put them to bed, remind them of all the positive things they have seen and done that day.

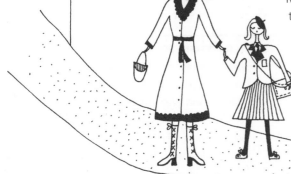

taming teens

961 GROW GRATITUDE

Help your family see the half-full glass (instead of the half-empty one) by making a habit of being grateful for at least one thing a day. Even if it's something as simple as 'I'm grateful the sun was shining', it will help them develop a positive outlook.

962 HELP THEM OPEN UP

Studies say that only about a quarter of kids discuss their worries with their friends. About the same number talk to their parents, but the majority try to deal with problems alone. Talk to your children often and help them open up to you. Kids in families who talk openly are more likely to turn to a parent first if faced with a crisis.

963 KEEP IT CHEAP

Don't worry if you haven't got lots of money to take your children on expensive outings. Research has shown that children are just as happy having a picnic in the park or simply hanging out at home with their parents – what they really need is for you to spend quality time with them.

964 TOO MANY NOS

Before you bite back with a 'no' to all your teenager's requests, examine why you want to say no and be open to discussion. If your teenager feels you are compromising, they will be more inclined to do the same.

965 GIVE PRAISE

You might assume your teenager doesn't now need or want your approval, but in fact they probably need it more than ever. Make sure they know you are proud of them.

966 KEEP RULES FLEXIBLE

Instead of setting out rigid rules with strict boundaries, try to keep them flexible so your teenager feels they have some say in the rule making and is more likely to obey.

967 ENJOY THE JOURNEY

Parents who give their teenagers their love, time, boundaries and encouragement to think for themselves may find that they actually enjoy this period in their kids' lives.

special needs

968 DON'T LAY BLAME

Many parents who have children with special needs feel anger or the desire to blame somebody (or themselves) for their child's condition. Understand that this is a very difficult time of adjustment and the acceptance process will take time.

969 REMEMBER YOUR OTHER KIDS

If you have a child with special needs, the temptation can be to give them lots of attention instead of your other children. Try to get some help organized so you can build in a morning or afternoon alone with each of your other children so they don't feel neglected.

970 BE A COUPLE

Having a child with special needs can put a lot of strain on marriages and partnerships and it's important to remember your relationship needs time too. Try to get out together once a month and find time to talk.

971 DO YOUR RESEARCH

There's a wealth of information available on the internet about most conditions and arming yourself with knowledge about your child's needs will put you in a stronger position to fight red tape and indifference.

972 CHANGE DOCTORS

If you don't feel your doctor or healthcare team is taking your child's problems seriously, don't be afraid to change to a different doctor. Set out your case clearly and avoid emotion.

973 BE A PUSHY PARENT

Parents of children with special needs have to speak out on their children's behalf even more than other parents. Often, being the best parent you can for your child means being pushy and asking questions.

974 GET SOME HELP

If you are the sole carer for a child or adult with special needs, make sure you take advantage of schemes available to give you a break. You'll be a better carer.

975 SEEK ADVICE

If you're concerned that your child may have special needs or you're worried about a specific condition, seek help as soon as possible. Many problems respond better to help when addressed at an earlier age.

976 DON'T TAKE NO FOR AN ANSWER

If there's something you think your child needs or would benefit from, fight for it and don't take no for an answer. Engage people to help you with your battles and give your child the best care you can.

menopause

977 KEEP A THERMOS

To help with night sweating, keep a thermos flask of ice water or an ice pack alongside your bed which you can use to help you cool down if you get hot in the night. At the onset of a hot flush, drink a glass of iced water or diluted fruit juice, which will help cool your body from the inside.

978 KNOW YOUR TRIGGERS

If you have hot flushes, mood swings, palpitations, panic attacks or other symptoms, take a pen and paper and write down what you were doing, thinking, feeling, who you were with and what you ate or drank just before so you can identify patterns.

979 KEEP DOING KEGELS

Menopause is a really important time to keep doing your Kegel exercises (clenching and relaxing the pelvic floor muscles) to stop future urinary incontinence and uterine prolapse. Tighten, hold for a few seconds then slowly release. Work up to holding for 10 seconds at a time and performing a set of 10 at least three times a day.

980 ONE A DAY

Because your body systems change after menopause, it can make you more susceptible to clotting problems such as stroke and heart attack. Taking an aspirin a day (under doctor's supervision) could help reduce your risk.

981 JUNK THE JUNK

Processed foods, nicotine, caffeine and artificial sweeteners are no-nos for menopausal women as they can exacerbate symptoms like flushing and mood swings. Try to keep your blood sugar levels as constant as possible.

982 BE SWEET ENOUGH

Try cutting out the artificial sweetener aspartame, which is found in many low-fat products, cordials and other sweetened foods, and which some believe can make menopausal symptoms worse.

983 LAYER UP

Almost all women will experience some sort of hot flushing or sweating around menopause, so it's sensible to be prepared by dressing in layers so you can peel them off to cope with changes in your temperature.

984 GET GARLIC

If you don't like the taste of garlic, make sure you don't miss out on its beneficial anti-cancer and blood pressure effects by taking an odourless garlic supplement daily. Brassica vegetables like broccoli and cabbage can also have the same effect.

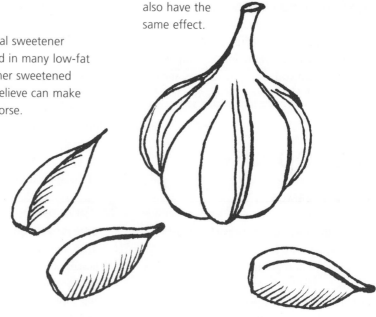

985 NATURAL FIBRES

To help reduce the intensity of hot flushes and let your skin breathe, make sure you use cotton sheets at night and try to choose natural fibres for the clothes you sleep in, lingerie and clothing that will touch your skin.

986 BE A MAG LADY

If you suffer menopausal palpitations, try taking 500 mg of magnesium, which is thought to help stop muscle flutters and spasms. Magnesium is also thought to help reduce migraines if taken early.

987 PACK IT IN

The quickest remedy for a hot flush is to use an ice pack or bag of frozen vegetables from your freezer. Place it on your neck, face, inner arms and wrists to help cool your blood.

988 FAN THE FLUSH

For travelling, use a mini portable fan to help you stay cool during hot flushes. Fan your face and hairline and even use a wet tissue or water spritzer to sponge your face first to enhance the cooling effect.

989 SPRINKLE CINNAMON

Adding cinnamon and ground flaxseed to your morning cereal can help your heart stay healthy, keep cholesterol low and reduce blood pressure, all of which are increased risks after menopause.

990 TAKE A STATIN

Menopausal women often suffer an increase in cholesterol as their oestrogen levels dip. As well as exercise and a healthy diet, your doctor may want you to take daily statins, which can help reduce cholesterol.

991 PLAIN SAILING

As women go through the menopause, they are more likely to develop heartburn, acid reflux and gallstones, so avoiding fried, rich, spicy foods and too much sugar is sensible.

992 SAY NO TO CHOCOLATE

It might seem like a feel-good food, but eating chocolate and any sweets during the menopause can actually make you feel bad by bringing on hot flushes, raising insulin levels and causing palpitations and anxiety.

993 DON'T GET ANGRY

Many women going through menopause report having uncontrollable anger and rage. Try to avoid situations that set you off and take lots of vitamin B to help tranquillize moods.

994 TURN OFF THE NEWS

Studies have shown that watching the local news is actually a contributor to high stress levels, which can make mood swings more likely. Do something relaxing instead.

995 GO LOW CARB

High-carbohydrate foods can cause hot flushes, anxiety and depression as well as elevating insulin levels, which can make symptoms worse. Also, your metabolism is likely to change at menopause, meaning you gain weight more easily.

996 SIP AWAY SICKNESS

A good remedy for the sickness often associated with menopause is to make up a drink with hot water, 2–3 tsp of lemon juice and, if you like, a little ginger. Sip slowly.

997 EDUCATE YOURSELF

One of the best ways to help yourself cope with the changes associated with menopause is to find out as much as you can about it and what to expect, which will help cut down anxiety. Research on the internet and talk to friends and family who have already gone through the process.

998 STOP BEING SUPERWOMAN

By the time many women reach the age of menopause, they are often relied on by many others – partners, parents, children, friends. Allow yourself to stop being superwoman for a while and look after yourself to help you through what is, after all, a perfectly natural process.

999 BOOST HORMONES NATURALLY

At menopause, oestrogen levels drop, which causes many of the unwanted symptoms. The soy isoflavones genistein and daidzein (mostly found as powders) are phyto-oestrogens which are thought to naturally mimic oestrogen to make menopause easier to cope with.

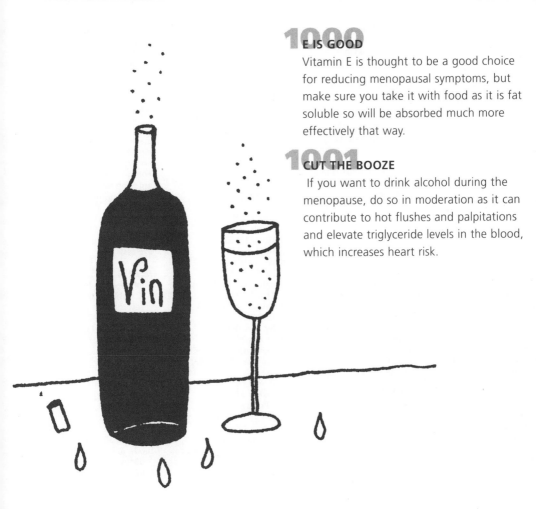

1990 E IS GOOD

Vitamin E is thought to be a good choice for reducing menopausal symptoms, but make sure you take it with food as it is fat soluble so will be absorbed much more effectively that way.

1991 CUT THE BOOZE

If you want to drink alcohol during the menopause, do so in moderation as it can contribute to hot flushes and palpitations and elevate triglyceride levels in the blood, which increases heart risk.